CW01376281

Yoga Magic

Copyright © Lyn Colenso 1999
ISBN No. 0-646-36318-2

All rights reserved.
Except under the conditions described in the Copyright Act 1968 of Australia and subsequent amendments, no part of this publication may be reproduced, stored in a retrieval system, or transmitted in any form or by any means, electronic, mechanical, photocopying, recording or otherwise, without the prior permission of the copyright owner.

Published in 1999 by
Novaprint Pty. Ltd.
41 Henderson Road, Clayton North 3168, Victoria
Printed in Australia by
Gunn & Taylor (Aust) Pty. Ltd.
Typeset by Susan Alford
Prepress by Resolution Imaging Pty. Ltd.
Bookbinding by M & M Binders Pty. Ltd.

Dedicated to the memory of
DOROTEA MANGIAMELE
Who taught me "To be with what is!"

With fondest memories and loving gratitude to Joy Spencer and Dr Raynor Johnson, who so generously gave me the tools to embark on this journey of the yoga.

With the greatest love to Nola Day, Peter Hockey, Wendy and David Bradtke, for sharing with me a passion for the yoga and the dance. I thank my dear friends Don, Jan and Gwen for their constant love and encouragement.

Special thanks to Annie, Bridget, Angie, Jessica, Charlotte, Zara, Emma Rose, and Dale for being such keen and appreciative students (and also for those hours spent taking those wonderful photos!).

Guru is a word which means "dispeller of darkness". This being the case, I must thank my husband, Nev, and my children, Maedy and Jonathan, who have been undoubtedly the greatest gurus ... I love you!

And to all those precious dancing children ... You are the future and you are what it is all about!

LYN COLENSO

"God give me grace to accept with serenity the things that cannot be changed, courage to change which should be changed, and the wisdom to distinguish the one from the other."

Reinhold Niebuhr

INDEX

1	Restraints
5	Observances
7	Reincarnation
9	Body of Light
19	The Opposites
23	Nature Says It All
31	Transience and Balance
37	The "Christ" Connection
43	The Serpent Power
45	Relationship and Solitude
47	The Postures, The Breathing, The Feeling
69	Meditation Plus Relaxation Equals Healing
73	The Dance of the Yoga

AUTHOR'S NOTE

Like a constant annoying little nudge, life has time and time again said to me in the depths of silence "you must write about IT". Time and time again I have ignored the nudge, with the usual justifications ...

But ... but ... by what authority do I claim enough knowledge to write this book? I don't have any qualifications in the vast and complex areas of psychology and philosophy. It seems to me that authors are those wonderfully talented people from some higher dimension of being that I could never aspire to reach.

And yet the thing I wish to share with the world most is my greatest passion ... YOGA. I want everyone to know how even after nearly 30 years it still comes up with something new, challenging, creative and transforming for me.

Of course during my journey through yoga and dance which began in 1971, I buried my head in countless books from Satyananda, Yogananda, Kriyananda, Muktananda (I lovingly call that my "Ananda" period – Ananda means bliss) right through to modern day masters like Deepak Chopra and Desikachar. Along the way I have struggled to digest the Yoga Sutras, the Bhagavad-Gita, and yet adored the simplicity of truth in such timeless inspired poetry as Kahil Gibran's "The Prophet", Rabindranath Tagore's "Gitanjali", and Edwin Arnold's "Light of Asia".

I sought gurus here, there, and everywhere until I finally discovered I was my own "guru". I called that my circuitous journey.

And yet it has been the practice of this YOGA itself that I find so amazing. Its strengths and yet its humility ... its ability to transform consciousness even in what seems to me now only a few moments.

I have taught this beautiful yoga ... postures (asanas), breathing practices (pranayamas), relaxation (nidra), meditation (dhyana) and the creative dance that is born of the yoga, for over 25 years. What I have found so intriguing and fascinating is how the postures can actually change a person's attitude towards themselves and towards life.

Most students of the yoga are seeking the benefits derived from physical suppleness, healthier, deeper breathing, and relaxation to balance a busy lifestyle. Some are there to heal their sick, tired bodies, learn how to correct bad posture, or to deal with an aching back or a broken heart. Mothers-to-be come to prepare positively for a more relaxed attitude to childbirth.

Of course all these things are important to quality of life. But I have actually experienced first hand how powerful these practices can be to really change areas of personality that you could normally find impenetrable. Little do yoga students realise the transformation they are embarking upon.

I have seen arrogance melt into humility ... conceit dissolve into compassion ... self-righteousness and martyrdom transform into uplifted energetic achievement. Maybe this is the true alchemy ... what is meant by changing base metal into gold (symbolically).

I have watched self-consciousness become super confident, indifference become efficient, selfishness become considerate, competitiveness become co-operative, fear become courageous, weakness become strong.

Even more exciting was the discovery of that which is truly sacred, magical, spiritual in every facet of life. I believe in maybe my over-the-top idealistic way, that such an expanded awareness has the potential to change the consciousness of the entire planet. Perhaps the rest of the universe knows the answers and is just patiently waiting for us to catch it up.

This is the yoga I discovered ... I gave it the name Bhava, which means "feeling", and I long to share it with you.

Lyn Colenso
Principal of The Bhava Centre,
Warrandyte, Victoria

FOREWORD

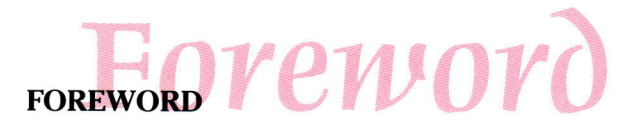

There are those of us who believe we are what we are … We inherit our nature, our attitudes, our physical genetics from our parents and those before. We are conditioned into certain cultural traits through early years into a particular way of living and thinking and we justify ourselves by believing all of these circumstances make up what we really are, and nothing in the world can change that.

YOGA begs to differ.

YOGA says you have a choice.

We have all heard the expression "you are what you eat" and/or "you are what you think". Yoga goes one further and says "you are your posture".

Our posture is what we portray to the outside world. It carries with it a particular attitude and it gives us a specific feeling towards that attitude. All it needs is an expanded awareness on our part to discover it for ourselves and then we can stay with it or change it.

Let's use FOOD as an example we can all relate to. We have the freedom to change our eating habits and acquire new and exciting tastes. We can choose to eliminate particular foods which were once part of our daily life, but now we know are harmful to our well being. We can enhance our taste experience by adding foods from other cultures, and in such a way we become different, even more colourful vibrant people. Of course we have every right to choose to remain locked into the eating habits we have always known and with which we feel safe. One choice could need an adventurous spirit but may enrich one's life, whilst the other would mean safety, predictability, and traditional values.

It is the same with posture. Most of us are locked into certain attitudes and expressions as if they were pre-conceived and placed in the blueprint of our beings. In most cases we take these attitudes for granted and even consider that we are "right" in our ways and everyone else is "wrong".

But the yoga suggests that there is no right and wrong, and the Bhava approach to yoga goes one step further to suggest it is more to the point that just as we can have the opportunity to taste a huge variety of foods in our own personal diet, so we have the choice of experiencing and developing a great many facets to our personality through posture. With awareness we can discover those attitudes that cause us pain and grief, those attitudes which enhance our sense of well being, and then we can make our own choices. As we become more in tune so to speak, we can actually watch our posture, hence our attitude, and if it is not to our liking, alter it almost immediately just by changing what we portray through our body language.

Once we embrace and practice the multitude of posture choices we have in the Yoga we are opening ourselves to a whole range of attitudinal experience which can only create a rich and abundant life.

It means the cultivation of humility on one hand and dignity on the other ... compassionate understanding and yet wise detachment ... surrender and acceptance blended with courage and strength. It means we can add to the rich tapestry of life many, many more coloured threads of actual individual experience.

We have all heard the expression "where there is light, there is no darkness". That is what the yoga is all about ... opening up the self to the divine self which is pure light.

There is no yoga posture which invokes feelings of anger, hatred, or violence. There is no yoga posture that invokes despair and depression. Nor is there any posture in the yoga which promotes attitudes of arrogance, conceit or self-righteousness.

How wonderfully refreshing it is to REALISE that we do have a choice.

Restraints

We are told that many thousands of years ago in India there arose amongst the sages of the time a practice called yoga ... a profound science which if practised with dedication would lead the chela (pupil) towards a wondrous understanding of spirit.

Yoga is a Sanskrit word meaning union ... perhaps, in an all embracing sense, union of the body, mind, heart with spirit ... union of black and white, negative with positive ... union of man and woman. Whichever way one looks at it yoga was obviously to bring about change ... transformation in consciousness ... change in attitudes and responses to life ... explosive union that could actually in a huge variety of ways create "NEW LIFE".

This remarkable science born of a "looking within" had the ability to turn one's life completely around so to speak, and its magic is as real today as we approach the year 2000, as ever before.

It is often thought that yoga was linked to particular eastern religions such as Hinduism and Buddhism, but the sages despite religious dogma and ritual, knew its secret was universal consciousness ... a state of awareness that couldn't be contained within any "place" of worship ... temple, mosque, cathedral, etc. In fact it brought about a real understanding that the human body was in fact a "place of worship", our very own temple so to speak. It required simply the practice of the yoga to open the floodgates wide to spiritual understanding.

Practitioners discovered an awakening of creative energy (Prana) but with a sense of conserving that energy ... an overwhelming appreciation of the magical process of nature ... an ability to create beauty ... an inner contentment so remarkably interwoven with courage ... an acceptance of life unfolding like the petals of a flower ... a profound wisdom. Those who enjoyed such a connection with their inner self seemed in an uncanny but somehow natural way to attract people to them ... thirsty souls perhaps ... lost, disillusioned maybe ... searching souls hungry for answers. And so it was that there were teachers (gurus) and students (chelas). Perhaps it helps us to understand that it is the very same process behind each and every religious belief from the beginning of time ... the aspirant sits at the feet of the master, listens and learns ... the tiny child sits at the feet of the parent, and the school children sit at the feet of their loving teacher ... the evolutionary wheel turns.

Perhaps an answer lies in the universality of this ancient and yet so appropriately modern yoga which can dissolve the so totally inappropriate differences between humans upon our wonderful planet earth ... For here is a beautiful practice that does not in any way suggest that 'this is right' and 'that is wrong'. Right and wrong simply melt into oneness and become this moment ... perhaps that is LOVE ... true understanding.

So what does it ask of the practitioner this yoga? The ancient sages suggested that man's anguish and suffering was very much the result of his or her mind processes ... in other words we virtually in spirit create our own unique situation in life no matter what that should be. So firstly the yoga could provide a virtual "taming" of the mind by the process of dealing with and eliminating conflict. Certainly not as easy as it sounds, but one has to start somewhere.

It was suggested that the best thing was to live everyday life in such a way that one didn't create conflict (or karma). In other words one should take complete responsibility for the choices one makes.

The first step was a series of moral and ethical codes ... like rules by which one lives life:

1. Avoid violence in any shape or form (to others, oneself, the creatures, the earth). The result would be a conservation of anger which meant that gradually one would understand the power of anger and how it can be transformed into strength. It was suggested that the result of violence and anger attracts only more violence, destruction, heartbreak and pain.

2. Live one's life taking only one's "just deserts" that which is purely earned and deserved. In other words stealing anything whether it be money, possessions, property, opportunity, whatever, makes for deep seated guilt, which in turn creates in the offender mistrust and suspicion in return.

3. To speak absolute truth and beyond all else be true to oneself first, for deceit has the possibility of enormous escalation and repercussion. Who was it said "Oh, what a tangled web we weave when first we practise to deceive"?

4. Understand the sacred energy of sex … the self-same wondrous energy from which humankind creates itself … the sacred energy of procreation in every form of nature. Learn to be discerning in the expression of sexual love. Before sharing such a precious gift look to the heart first. The sages suggested that the vital life force (Prana) is replenished by love but depleted by lust. Perhaps to misuse such sacred energy could have far reaching repercussions in health and well being. Only the heart knows the answer … only the heart knows the mysteries.

5. Become aware of attachments … It was suggested that even as life gives to us our family, our friends, our loved ones, our homes, our possessions, our achievements, our health, our bodies … any obsession with holding onto and controlling these can cause us incredible anguish. Such possession, which is not always obvious, stifles the possibility for growth and change which is the natural law of the universe. Difficult as it seems, it is suggested we need to "let go" the controls and trust in the process of life and its transient nature.

Each of these codes is quite complex and obviously open to personal interpretation. It is uncanny how each of us can twist them around to suit ourselves only to find them facing us up front in every mirrored reflection. And so we begin to see the profound psychology of the yoga and this is only the beginning.

Observances

It is human nature no doubt that makes us hungry and thirsty ... natural instincts which determine our existence and our survival. It is also human nature that we experience fear and anxiety of anything that threatens our survival. Like building blocks one emotion builds upon the other and we find ourselves also experiencing anger, frustration, jealousy, greed. It is then that our see-saw of tension surges upwards. And when we feel we are losing or have already lost that which is precious in our lives, we then have emotions of despair and depression, and see ourselves as a victim of circumstances. Then the see-saw plummets downwards.

But the higher self watches the process from afar ... as we imagine in religious practices that God (or the Gods) watches us from on high ... from some distant cloud ... or some glorious heavenly place inhabited by angels. Through the ages people have had trouble understanding the higher self as being within them, hence the sense of separateness. But through the yoga perhaps we see it that gradually the vast distance between human basic nature and higher self diminishes. Maybe one could say yoga brings us closer to that part of us which responds to the mystery of stillness, that feels deep contentment, a sense of wholeness and fulfilment.

It could perhaps help to equate it to the vision of a loving parent quietly watching the constant antics of their small children ... and the whole scenario is within our individual unified self.

Our higher self is THAT peace, THAT stillness, THAT contentment. Is it any wonder the ancient masters of the yoga would repeat again and again "THOU ART THAT"? The same wise ones suggest that certain observances are of great benefit upon our personal journey towards realisation.

1. Cleanliness in every respect. Cleanliness of body, of eating and drinking habits, of thought, of motive, of environment.

2. Contentment ... to try as best one can despite normal desires and challenges, to be contented with self ... to periodically leave the demands of the day to discover that inner contentment.

3. Austerity ... to live a disciplined life as far as possible, which in turn creates self-respect and dignity. It must be pointed out however that austerity does not mean personal abuse or deprivation, but discipline where a loving attitude always prevails.

4. Self-study ... To take time to study oneself closely ... but not to the point of degradation or despair. Appreciate the qualities you see, but honestly acknowledge the weaknesses, the secret being to love the self for where it is regardless ... success or failure. It is important to realise we each have the possibility of beginning again and again. Remember that this very moment is the beginning of the rest of your life, the rest of your journey.

5. Surrender to the higher self ... We are encouraged in the yoga to discover the joy that comes through surrendering everything to "what is". It means to trust in a higher process ... an acceptance of things beyond our control. How often life astounds us. Situations change quite remarkably with very little effort on our part, and most times in a totally unpredictable way.

REINCARNATION

Quite apart from religious belief the sages suggest that the soul travels on a journey of many lifetimes ... each individual lifetime, no matter what the circumstances or environment, providing a unique opportunity to learn, to grow, in other words to evolve.

Lessons that have not been fully understood in one lifetime therefore need to be addressed in future lives ... hence the theory of karma. Karma could be explained as the natural law of the universe ... that each action in life brings about a certain result. Maybe such a theory helps us to understand more fully the adage ... "you get what you deserve from life".

If there is the remotest possibility that one reincarnates, it would follow that the subconscious mind is jam-packed with wondrous memories ... visions of beauty and ugliness ... places of joy and horror ... many, many cultures from all parts of our planet earth ... and even perhaps far beyond. You may have noticed how often when a person visits ancient places on the planet there is a sort of triggering of memory in a way that can be quite emotional at times ... as if discovering a deep connection inside to that particular place.

Perhaps our connection with different cultures has a marked effect on our tastes in music, art ... even to the planting of different exotics in our gardens. There is no denying that such a theory embraces a multi-cultural society and maybe someday a "global" family.

It would follow that each one of us could have experienced in past lives incredible feelings of despair and struggle, puffed up experiences of arrogance and self-righteousness, times of holding tyrannic power over others, balanced by times of victimisation. Deep in the recesses of our complex minds there could be the making of fantastic soap operas or even mini-series. Such a theory shows us where that drive comes from to write a novel, compose a symphony, paint a masterpiece, weave a tapestry, build a cathedral, or whatever.

Bhava yoga acknowledges this complex creative mind within each aspirant and dives right into its depth in every yoga session. Having awakened the possibilities of a vast imagination, it uses that same awareness to get in touch with the magical aspects that make up the physical being. The journey of the yoga helps the student to discover various layers of consciousness. Through the creative practice of postures the magic of the physical being is enhanced. One becomes aware of a life force the yogis of old called Prana ... without which there could be no life as we know it. Awareness of this Prana helps us to understand our "body of light" (or lightness) also realising that Prana is all pervading ... in earth, water, air, space and even beyond. Each one of us can actually learn how to use that Prana to increase our vitality, heal the body, and claim a rich and abundant life. It all begins with the creative imaginative mind.

When we practise the postures (asanas) of the yoga, the Bhava approach takes the practitioner to an awareness of a particular feeling and attitude that each posture brings about. Focussing the attention to such a feeling, locks it into the psyche. Prana (life force) is directed to the bodyform because of the focussing of the mind and it is that focussing that causes the remarkable attitudinal change.

After considerable practising of this approach to yoga, one begins to realise that they are capable of experiencing many very positive attitudes which in their own way produce a vast knowledge of life itself. Perhaps it is in a way a journey towards greater understanding, strength of character and wisdom.

BODY OF LIGHT

Once we discover for ourselves an awareness of an energy body or "body of light" … (the ancient yogis called it "Prana-Maya-Kosa" – life force-veil-body) we come to understand something that eastern medicine has recognised for thousands of years. Let us say that all of the thousands upon thousands of tiny nerves that make up our nervous system are channels or pathways carrying Prana or life force invisibly around our body. The yogis called these channels nadis (the Chinese – meridians).

The ancient masters suggest there are 72,000 nadis in our body of light, the most important being a channel following the spinal cord – from the base right through to the top of the skull, the fontanel area. This channel was called Sushumna … and could be related to the central nervous system.

The parasympathetic and sympathetic nervous systems were not ignored because these two major channels of life force were said to travel in relationship with the spine … Ida nadi on the left and Pingala nadi on the right. Ida and Pingala flow with Prana commencing at the base of Sushumna and crisscrossing Sushumna at various points along the way completing their journey at a point at the back of the eyebrow centre, where all three nadis become one in Sushumna where the Prana then continues its journey up to the top of the head and even beyond.

If you are feeling lost by now hang in there because the practice of the yoga will reveal all as your creative imaginative mind is awakened and focussed.

The incredibly exciting thing is that where Ida and Pingala cross over through Sushumna there are said to be powerful energy centres (the masters called these centres Chakras). Maybe it helps to think of power lines and where they come together at various points, there is a power station storing and distributing more electrical energy.

The uncanny thing is that medical science today confirms that in the physical anatomy at each so-called energy centre (Chakra) suggested by the yogic masters, there is a ductless gland which is part of the amazing endocrine system and therefore part of that magical world of hormones in our physical bodies. Remember the Chakras are of the body of light (etheric or pranic body) ... the glands are in the physical body, which could not function without life force. Chakra is a Sanskrit word meaning wheel – it is said to spin and spiral like a wheel of light.

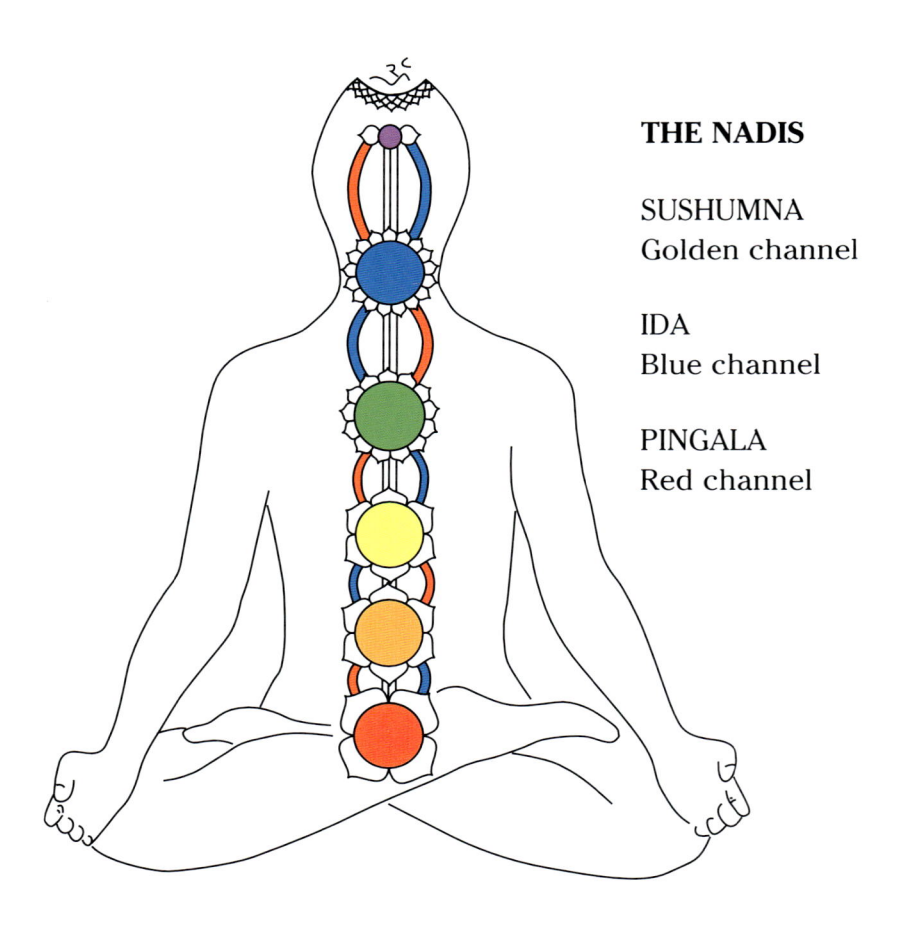

THE NADIS

SUSHUMNA
Golden channel

IDA
Blue channel

PINGALA
Red channel

THE CHAKRAS

SAHASRARA – Spirit

AJNA – Mind

VISHUDDHI – Space

ANAHATA – Air

MANIPURA – Fire

SWADHISTHANA – Water

MOOLADHARA – Earth

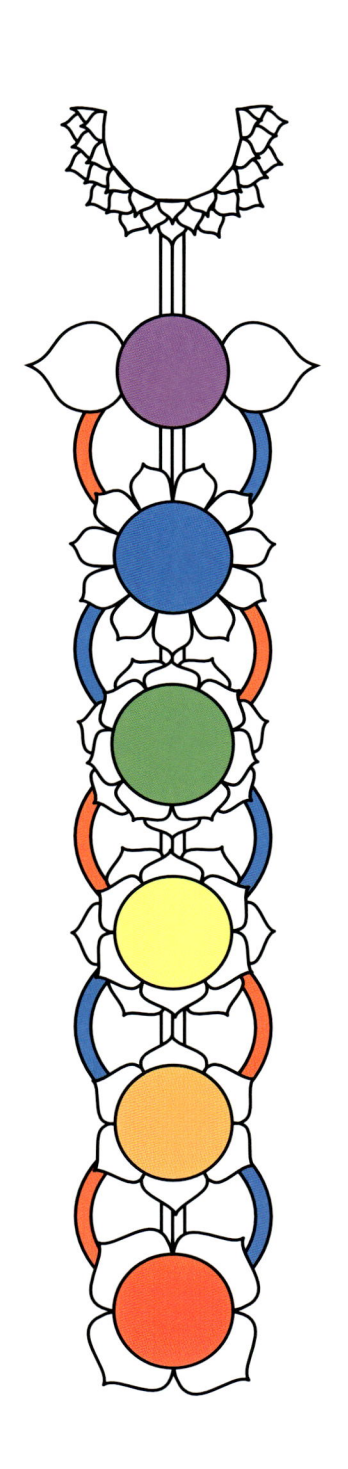

II

Let's have a look at these Chakras from a Bhava yoga viewpoint:

THE EARTH CENTRE *(Mooladhara Chakra)* is at the base of the spine and relates to the sexual organs – the centre of the powerful energy of reproduction/procreation. Yoga practices help us to focus on the pelvic floor to enhance our sexuality and feel our strong connections to the earth – awareness of Mooladhara helps us to keep our feet firmly planted on the earth at all times and face up to our responsibilities. The drumming musics of the primitive indigenous people are very earth centred. Visualise bright red (scarlet) at this centre. The yogis used as a symbol of the earth Chakra the elephant, but an appropriate symbol could be a solid gold block or cube like a solid gold ingot.

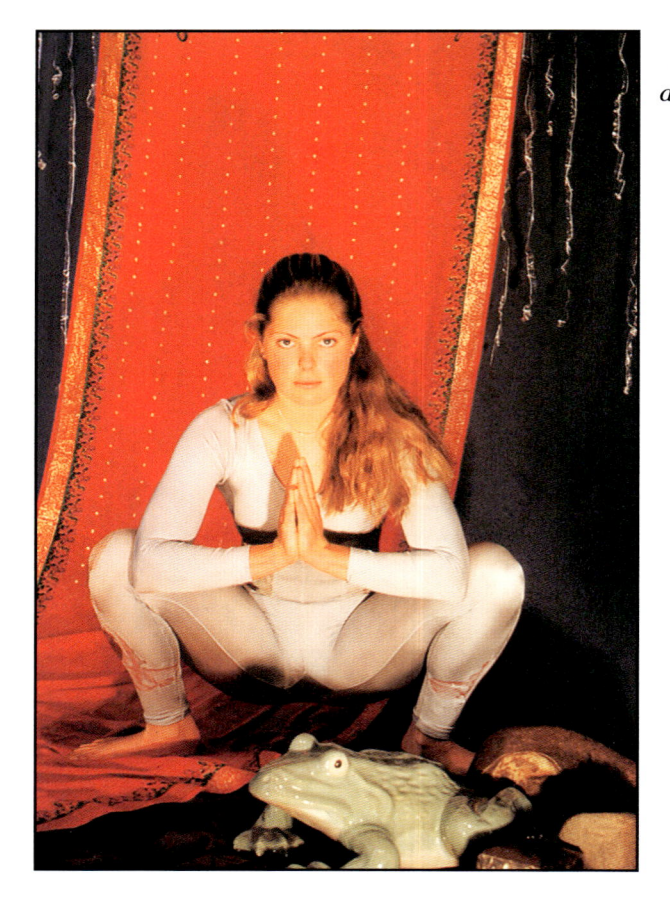

NAMASKARA
(Squatting Posture)
awakens Mooladhara

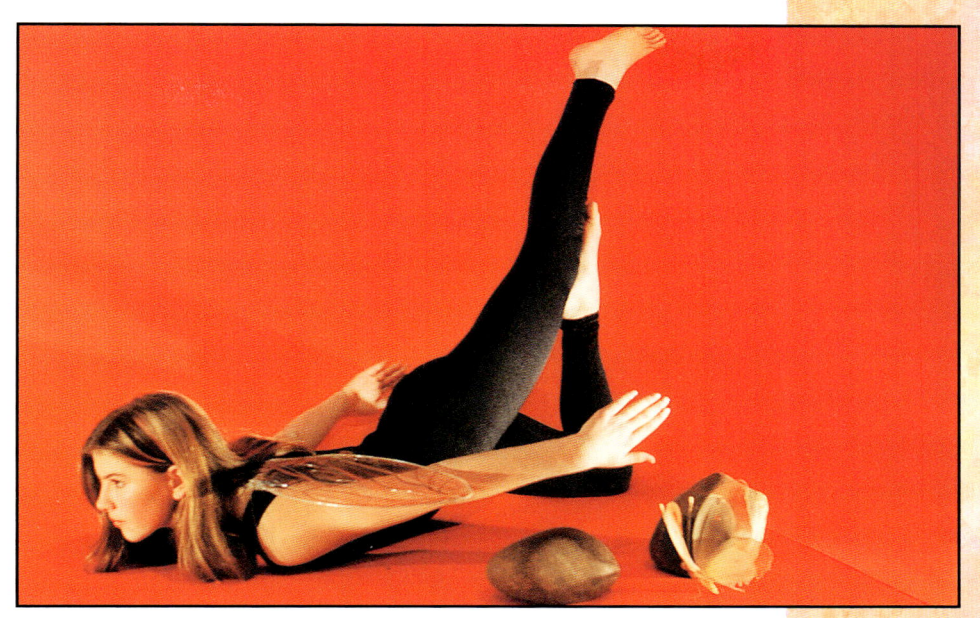

SALABHASANA (Flying Locust Posture) awakens Swadhisthana

THE WATER CENTRE *(Swadhisthana Chakra)* is in the pelvic region and lumbar spine. It relates to the adrenal glands and is involved in the elimination process of the body. Consider the position of the uterus in the female body and the soft warm fluid that supports the unborn child in the water centre. Awareness of Swadhisthana within the yoga practice creates an ability to flow more with life like the tides of the ocean, or the journey of a river to the sea. It helps to awaken flexibility towards life and self. Visualise the colour orange in the centre of the pelvic region and an inverted half moon floating on its back like a quaint little boat or barge floating on quiet waters. Water has the ability to find its own level and settle very close to the earth, like the lake in the valley.

THE FIRE CENTRE *(Manipura Chakra)* This is said to be in the solar plexus behind the navel and relates to the pancreas within the physical body. Its energy has to do with digestion and assimilation of food (nourishment) in the system. Postures which focus on Manipura create an incredible amount of physical energy and vitality – like igniting a wondrous fire of enthusiasm inside. It is a centre of heat and greatly aids physical circulation, boosting inner emotional strengths as well. Visualise a pot-bellied stove inside ... the colour bright golden yellow like the burning sun, and use the vibrant sun as your symbol at the solar plexus, the sun centre.

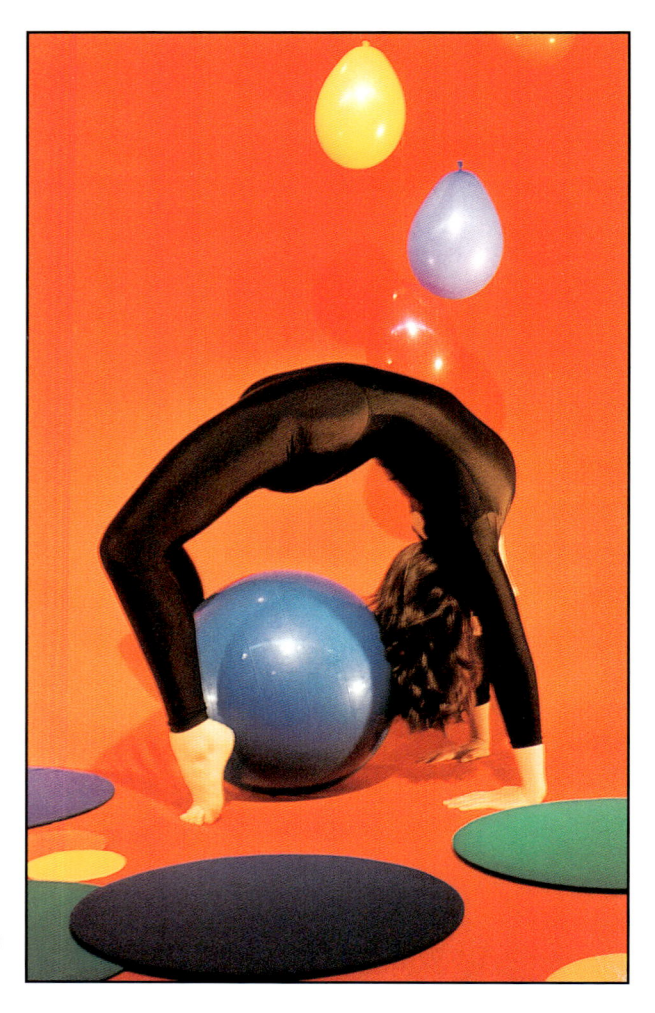

*CHAKRASANA
(Wheel/Bridge Pose)
awakens Manipura*

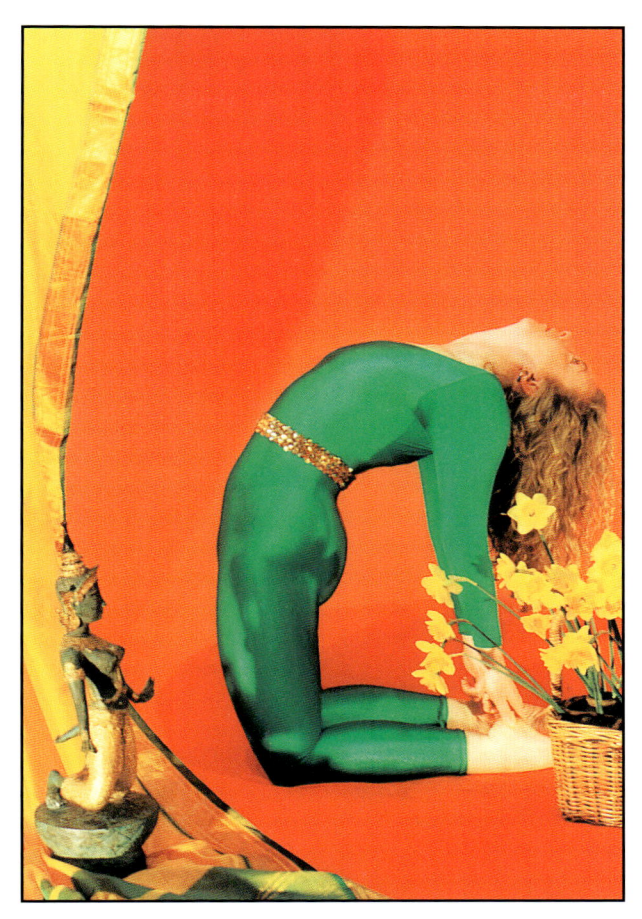

*USHTRASANA (Camel Pose)
awakens Anahata*

THE HEART CENTRE *(Anahata Chakra)* This is the centre of air – the air we breath – it is in the centre of the chest cavity – the position of the thymus gland in our physical body. Its energy is to do with the lungs and heart. Postures focussing on Anahata produce beautiful feelings of love in a totally selfless, unconditional, all encompassing way. It reveals to the practitioner a wonderful sense of self-worth and glowing confidence which begins to reveal itself through posture and radiance. Joy and light-heartedness are its gifts. To fly like a bird ... to glide like an eagle are the feelings of heart centre movement. Visualise jewel green in Anahata like an emerald glistening in light. An appropriate symbol could be a six pointed star of light studded with emeralds.

THE THROAT CENTRE *(Vishuddhi Chakra)* This is the centre of ether or space, that which is lighter than air, and is related to the thyroid gland. Its energy is to awaken our communication skills in life particularly through our voice ... not just speaking clearly and confidently, but also using our voice as an instrument of music and joy through singing and chanting. Postures focussing on Vishuddhi heighten our awareness greatly and seem to transform us in remarkable and positive ways to a greater appreciation of the beauty of life. Visualise a magical sapphire blue lagoon at Vishuddhi and allow yourself to dive deep into its bluenesss ... the symbol being a golden ring of light representing a "gateway" through which we can move into even higher levels of consciousness.

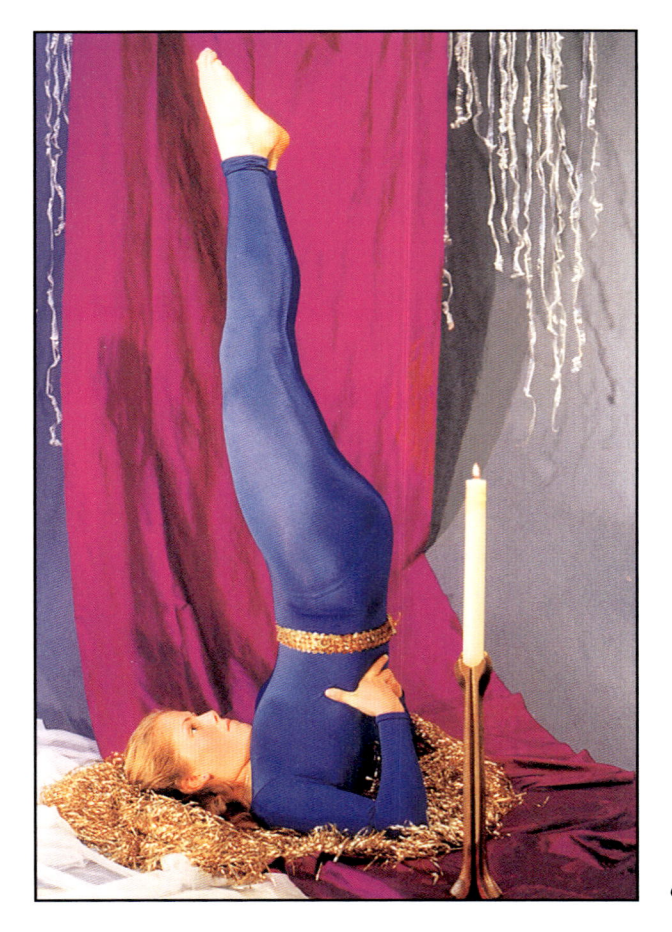

*SARVANGASANA
(Shoulder Stand)
awakens Vishuddhi*

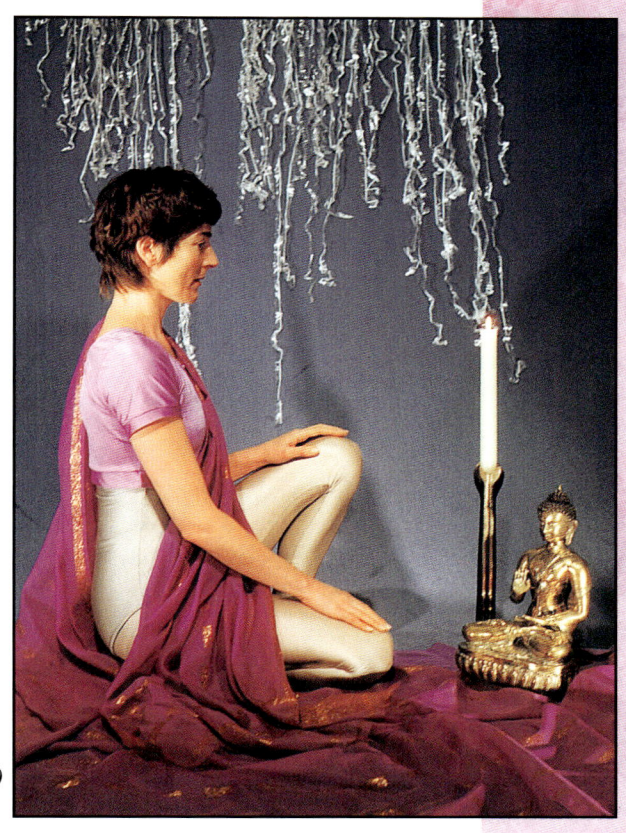

TRATAK (Candle Gazing) awakens Ajna

THE EYEBROW CENTRE *(Ajna Chakra)* The point between the eyebrows is like another "gateway" to the amazing depths of the mind. Could it be that this is what is meant by "the window to the soul"? Ajna has been called the third eye because this is the point where we visualise, we dream and we use our creative imagination. This is the point where we direct our mind to focus. Ajna's energy works closely with the pituitary and pineal glands distributing vital hormones and balancing the endocrine system. Practices that focus on Ajna bring about clear logical thinking, vivid imagination, and an ability to see one's purpose or direction in life. Focussing on Ajna helps us to be decisive, to gain a clear direction to our individual purpose, and certainly holds the magical key to unlocking a treasure trove of self-made opportunity. Visualise a violet mist between the eyebrows allowing it to slowly deepen to a rich purple at the back of the head. An inspiring symbol in the eyebrow centre could be an eternal flame burning.

SAHASRARA *(The Thousand Petalled Lotus)* This is more of an infinite experience of light rather than an actual Chakra which is a wheel of light. The ancient yogis explain it as a pure white lotus flower opening its thousands of beautiful petals to reveal a golden centre ... its wonderful fragrance all around ... giving of its beauty and yet receiving constant light from the sun above, an even higher source of energy. Focussing on Sahasrara will happen as a natural consequence of the awakening of each of the previous Chakras and can happen spontaneously in meditation (sitting). The experience brings about deep contentment, inner peace and wisdom, and is the state of bliss or ecstasy the yogis call Samadhi. Its colour is pure white light, the symbol of course the thousand-petalled white lotus with a pure gold centre.

If you have been really taking in the colours of the Chakras on the way, you will see that we have the colours of a rainbow ... red, orange, yellow, green, blue, violet. The pure white is of course that which is beyond the rainbow. The rainbow inside the mind – Wow! Consider how, even as a tiny child you delighted at the magic of a rainbow ... moving your very spirit with delight ... and now you have a link to that mystery ... inside and outside are obviously one and the same.

Also notice the elements connected with the Chakras ... the very same elements which are imperative to our physical existence and survival ... Earth, Water, Fire, Air, Space, Mind and Spirit.

The yoga goes so far as to suggest that it can weave the magic of the colours and the elements into a rich tapestry of oneness.

THE OPPOSITES

Think about a magnet with negative and positive fields ... opposite energy fields attracting, like energy fields rejecting. You might say the entire universe stays together in such a way. So is it any wonder that nature has created each one of us with our very own opposites so that we might be in some sort of balance with life?

The yogis knew thousands of years ago the mystery of each of us, regardless of gender, having a feminine and a masculine side to our being and even to our personality. When we tip the scales we find ourselves favouring one aspect of our being way over the other. For example if we favour the masculine side developing too much assertiveness, strength, dominance, adamant behaviour and the like, we may discover we have neglected the side of our nature that is compassionate, understanding and gentle. If however we focus predominantly on our feminine side developing a loving, nurturing, sympathetic nature, we might find that we lack certain strengths needed not to compromise ourselves, and be taken advantage of. It is a very delicate balance we discover in the practice of the yoga and one that should perhaps be looked at clearly and honestly.

It is well acknowledged these days that we have what is called the left side of the brain and the right side. Teachers are encouraged to give their students from a very early age not just knowledge and mental exercise to awaken the intellect, but also artistic and creative activities to awaken the imagination. We live in a time zone unfortunately where a large majority of children and adults are driven to succeed and discouraged to just BE. "Compete or fail" is the motto, and hence we have imbalance within human beings causing dissatisfaction, depression and general unhappiness. The ancient masters taught the balance of "being as well as doing".

So how do we correct the imbalance? We come back to those Nadis we previously spoke of ... Ida and Pingala. Ida, we are told, represents the feminine aspects of our nature i.e. loving attitude, nurturing, understanding, compassion, forgiveness, gentility. It follows that Pingala is the masculine counterpart, awakening strength of character, courage, assertiveness, confidence and the ability to face up to responsibilities.

So in the well balanced individual (male or female) we have Ida and Pingala flowing in harmony, like two beautiful rivers of light, their perfect dance crisscrossing Sushumna at the Chakras (wheels of light). But as most of us are far from perfect and perhaps one side

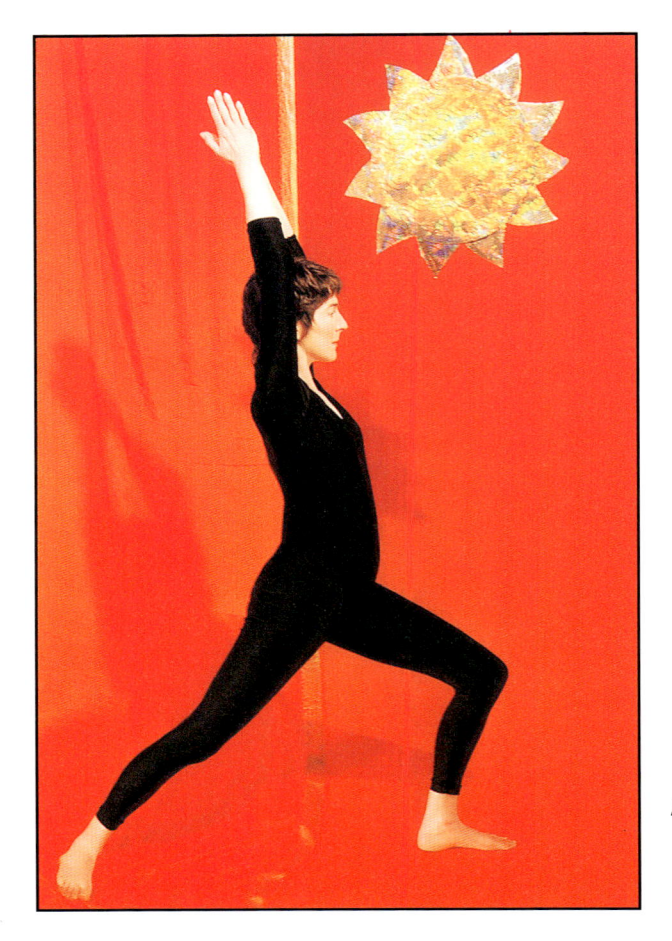

SURYASANA ... THE SUN POSE
Masculine/positive aspect invoking a sense of purpose, stability and responsibility

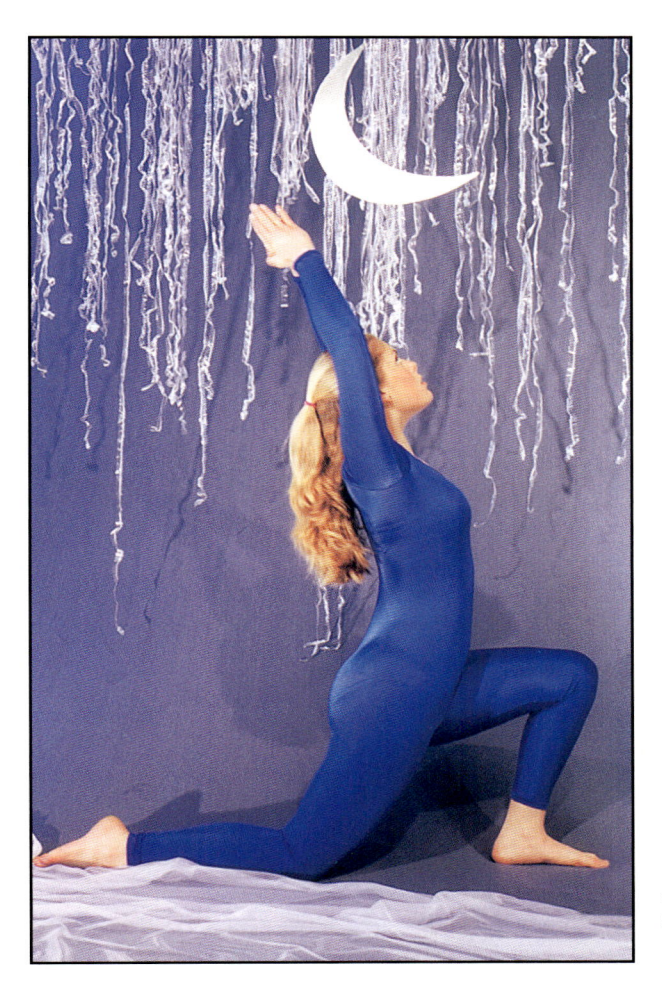

*CHANDRASANA
... The Moon Pose
Feminine/receptive aspect
awakening suppleness and
grace, flexibility and ease*

SURYA/CHANDRA united become the oneness we call YOGA.

is a little sluggish, we can learn from the various practices of the yoga just how to stimulate these Nadis and awaken whichever side of our being is lacking. For without that balance we are a little lop-sided in our view on life, and will find it very difficult to realise true happiness and inner peace.

Think back on the classic fairytales of old. Symbolic stories would tell of a beautiful princess or delicate maiden awaiting the love of a handsome courageous prince, or brave knight on his white charger. It seemed that without the other one could only be half alive. Only with a magical kiss could they unite and live happily ever after. The Bhava way of approaching yoga goes so far as to call the Nadis, Princess Ida and Prince Pingala and shows the magical way their courtship leads to "married bliss", in other words, perfect union (which is what the word yoga means). It is a slow and steady journey but the magical fairytale is real within each of us.

When the "dance" of the opposite energies becomes harmonious we feel for ourselves that change in consciousness – for some it seems almost miraculous – but it means we are slowly becoming more spiritually aware. In other words we are making a connection with our spirit ... our source ... our higher self.

The heightened awareness we experience gives us a greater appreciation of beauty, of love, of wonder, of natural miracles. Magic is revealed in the mere opening of the petals of a flower, the sunlight glistening like a diamond in a tiny dewdrop, the music of the lapping lilting seashore. We are connecting with a vast natural healing energy so we begin to feel more alive and alert. We are embarking on a profound journey towards wholeness ... towards health, physically and mentally ... towards holiness ... towards oneness with WHAT IS!

NATURE SAYS IT ALL

What does a butterfly contribute to the planet? What is the purpose of a flower? Why do we share our planet with all sorts of creatures?

When you consider the caterpillar it seems to spend its life greedily consuming every green leaf in sight. At some point it is guided instinctively to secrete the finest of silken threads to enfold itself into a magical cocoon of stillness ... absolute stillness ... where in obviously the most perfect retreat from the outside space, protected from cold, heat and/or predators, this peculiar creature transforms. It changes not just in consciousness but in physical form, to become an exquisite butterfly or moth – a creature not of the earth, but of the air – a creature so fine, with translucent colourful wings, that cannot only flutter but actually fly. The butterfly never fails to delight tiny children and adults alike.

Without the use of any words at all, nature is showing us through the metamorphosis of the butterfly just how each one of us is also on a similar spiritual journey and no matter how long it takes we will and can transform. (It is not surprising that Bhava Yoga chooses the butterfly as its symbol.)

Consider how it is with the flowers, whether they be wildflowers, shrubs, trees, perennials, bulbs, whatever. In order to achieve beautiful blossoms there needs to be a full cocktail of the elements – earth, water, sunlight, air and that magic beyond. Doesn't it always amaze you that from that tiny seed, that dull brown bulb, or prickly dead branches, come the most magnificent growth, flowers, roses, daffodils, camellias, magnolias, daisies, gerberas, lilies, violets ... the list goes on and on.

O tiny bulb, did you ever know the secret of your soul?
Did you dream day by day, that your dreary shell
Hid a beauty beyond compare?
Was it by chance you were embedded in damp, warm soil,

*And slowly there you found hidden joy
In spreading roots and shooting out
Pulled between the earth and the sun
Exploding with gratitude!*

*Did you ever know what lay ahead as leaves and
stem began to form
And what is this "bud" which builds up day by day
Like a storehouse of energy, bulging at the seams
Bursting into the yellow joy, you teased me so ...
And were you impatient as I, 'til the petals opened wide
To release the golden trumpet, ringing out
that spring is nigh?*

*O daffodil, so proudly you stand,
Bouncing rays of sunshine into the hearts of men
Giving and receiving, perfection is yours.
Tell me, O tiny bulb, did you ever know
The storehouse of beauty you contained?
Did you ever guess for a moment why you were here?*

Flowers are so unique in colour and petals, and even more amazing each variety has its own individual fragrance. To conceive a world without flowers is unheard of, such is their ability to lift our consciousness as human beings. As we delve deep into the ancient cultures we realise more and more the healing properties of many flowers and herbs, not to mention their fragrances ... the flower essences and fragrant oils that enhance our lives, healing and relaxing our minds.

The yogis took as their symbol of the unfolding consciousness of us human beings, the lotus blossom. The journey of the lotus begins deep in the mud at the bottom of the pond. As its roots go deep down to feed from the earth, its shoot travels up from the earth into the water. When you consider it, the experience of water is a different texture to the earth, but at the bottom of the pond is still quite mirky. You could say "vision" would be a little cloudy. As the lotus plant grows upwards instinctively towards light, the water begins to become cleaner until it becomes crystal clear near the surface. (As we grow in our individual consciousness we find things become a little clearer. It is interesting to consider that the water is naturally clearer at the surface ... the lotus has, however, to grow to realise that clarity.)

The lotus bud is well formed by the time it breaks through the surface of the water into the air ... and still the plant grows completely beyond the water before the petals begin to unfold. That magical unfolding of beauty and fragrance reveals a rich golden centre like a miniature sun. Its blossoming is a triumph of perfection and brilliance. A great understanding of the natural law of giving and receiving is realised, as the lotus gives so openly of its wondrous beauty (its heart) to the world, and receives joyfully the light and energy from the sun (universal love) in return. It is truly a symbol of generosity and a rich and abundant life (a full blossoming).

The yogic masters were so in awe of the lotus blossom that it became their absolute symbol of unfolding consciousness at all levels of awareness ... each of the Chakras (psychic energy centres) had their very own lotus symbol, and as depicted in each and every statue of Buddha, a pure white thousand-petalled lotus represents enlightenment (self-realisation). Consider the beauty of thousands of pure white petals continually unfolding in a never ending experience of beauty and fragrance within your own being, and allow your mind to dive deep into the centre of such a vision. You will probably never be the same again.

It has been suggested through the ages that the masters attained their wisdom and inspiration towards the creation of the various yoga practices of Asanas (postures) and Pranayamas (breathing techniques) by close observation of the creatures and their attitudes. The incredible realisation is that as human beings we are each one of us a cocktail of all of the creatures in a way ... in attitude, in postures, in movement, in appetite, in instinct. But, of course, we have a few added features ... desire, intellect, creative mind, freedom of choice, and most importantly, LOVE.

The elephant, noted for strength, endurance and longevity, was observed as breathing slowly and deeply, being steady and predictable. The tiny field mouse on the other hand, was observed as fearful and timid, with quick shallow breathing indicative of hypertension and short lifespan. The dog (man's best friend) has qualities of loyalty and protection. The members of the cat family like the lion and the tiger are regal creatures combining dignity and suppleness.

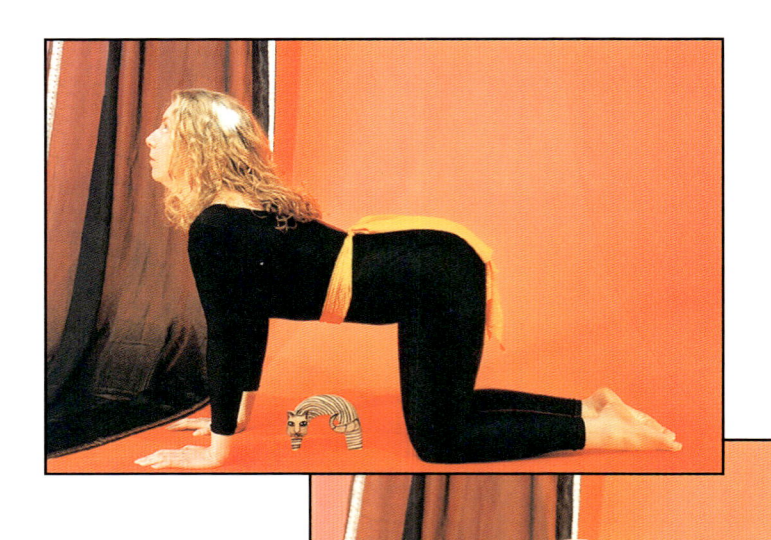

MARJARIASANA (THE CAT) Movements between hunching (like an angry cat) and arching help the practitioner to experience the suppleness and sensuality of the spine

The cobra snake rises out of the earth and with no resistance of movement opens its hood to the universe, in other words opening body, mind, heart to spirit. The camel has grace and patience and a large heart, whilst the crocodile waits and watches and never misses an opportunity when it comes close. The fish breathes through its gills and moves without the use of limbs. The monkey is so flexible it seems made of rubber. The frog is a creature of the earth and the water, a creature of soft jelly as if there are no bones inside. The bird is perfectly balanced on the branch before it learns to fly, and the eagle is completely focussed as it glides as if motionless in a never ending spiral.

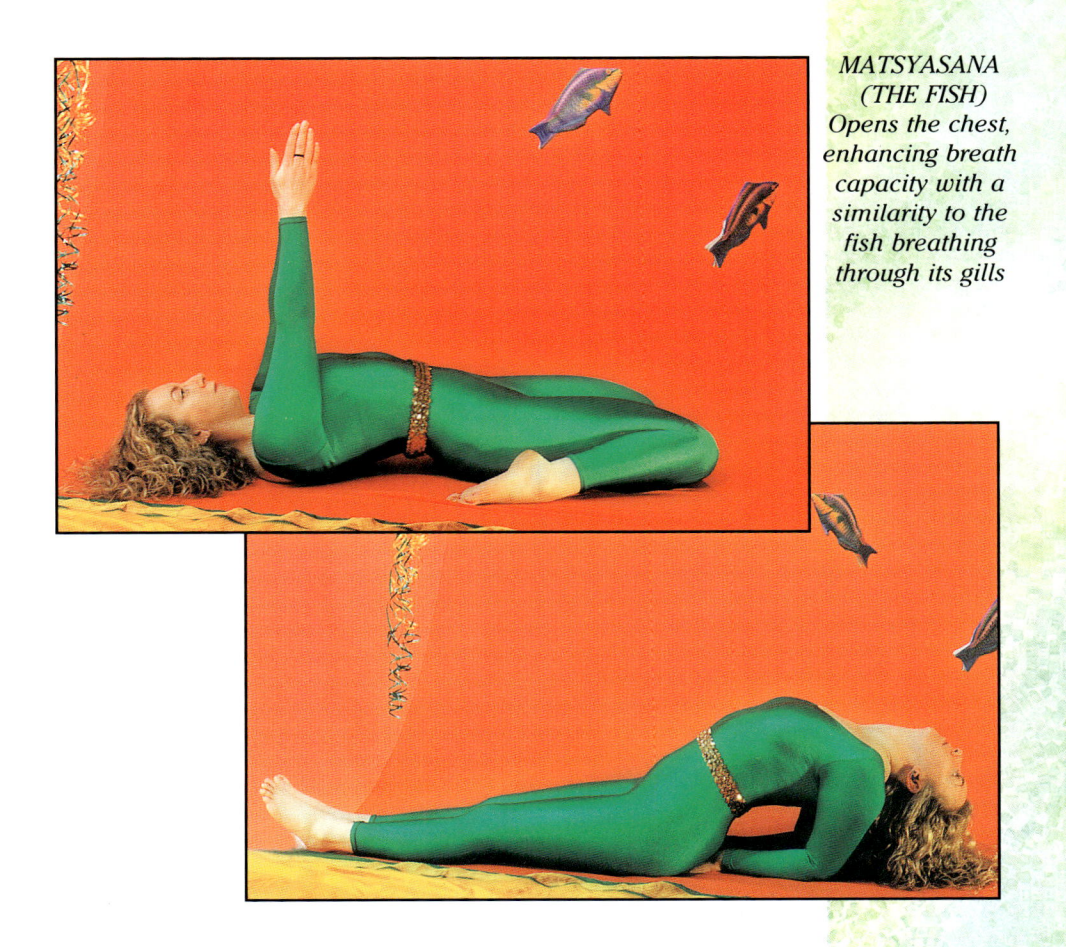

MATSYASANA (THE FISH) Opens the chest, enhancing breath capacity with a similarity to the fish breathing through its gills

The locust is quick and sharp, whilst the lizard basks in the warm sunshine relaxed with the earth. The swallow swoops and dives and the turtle has the strongest shell on its back. The snail glides in and out of its spiralling home making silver trails upon the earth.

The indigenous peoples echo the sacred connections with the creatures. The Australian Aboriginal people have wondrous legends of all the birds, insects and animals with which they share the land. They seem to have an understanding that there is a part of their being which relates to each and every creature ... the kangaroos, wallabies, emus, brolgas, snakes, lizards. Their very existence depended of course on bush tucker, and each creature devoured was said to connect with their very own spirit. The wonderful stories of the Rainbow Serpent show us the magical influence of colours within the mind of the primitive and yet so intuitive peoples.

The Native American Indians were incredibly connected with the animal kingdom. Their totems usually represented a combination of maybe four or five creatures placed one on top of the other as if depicting the integration of those animals' qualities and attitudes in the make up of an individual chief, medicine man, or the whole tribe. The wolf, the eagle, the mountain lion, the deer, the crow, the owl, were just a few.

The Druids of old in Europe were in awe of the creatures and felt blessed by the gods when "visited" by one. The cow represented fertility, the bull – virility and abundance of life. The fox depicted cunning, the swan – grace and beauty, the stag – pride and independence. The hawk was said to be that part of us that is noble – the goose was a symbol of procreation and parenting (hence the expression – mother goose). The bear represented strength and sovereignty, the otter – playful and filled with joy. This is just to name a few. The Druids also conjured up in their minds powerful and fierce creatures called dragons, as being those parts of our psyche which need to be challenged and overcome. To slay dragons was to destroy weaknesses and destructive attitudes. However often a dragon was depicted as a guardian protecting a deep cave which was filled with precious gems (perhaps the cave of our heart which is where the real treasure can be found!).

Perhaps the eagle, representing intelligence and courage would be a welcome archetype when faced with a dragon or two!

Yoga awareness helps you to notice the creatures which seem part of your everyday life. For instance there may be blue wrens dancing in your garden, or rabbits raiding the vegie patch, or a pair of eagles that you often watch spiralling overhead, a horse you know quite well, a friendly dove or magpie, a possum who scampers across your roof at night, a tiny field mouse who keeps turning up like the proverbial bad penny, and you just haven't got the heart to kill it, a sneaky fox who seems to come closer to your house than normal, a special faithful dog who snuggles up against your feet, a particular cat with whom you seem to continually make eye contact.

Perhaps you will become more aware of that mopoke owl you hear at night or the squawking cockatoos, the little echidna searching for honey ants. You may even be lucky enough to know kangaroos or wallabies, or work with animals in a sanctuary, a zoo, or an animal refuge. If you have the opportunity of connecting with farm life, take a moment or two to really look into the eyes of the beautiful cows full of milk and nurturing … the sheep, the ducks, the geese, the hens.

You may be experiencing a very important part of your "being"!

Transience

TRANSIENCE AND BALANCE

It was Buddha, the Enlightened One, who apparently was most disturbed when he first became aware of the transience of life. Buddha was said to have begun his life as Prince Gautama, born to a Maharaja and his Queen and he was protected all through his childhood behind the walls of the royal palace.

His father did everything he could to only reveal beauty and love to the little boy, but the story is told of the first time the prince, when learning to shoot an arrow, killed a bird ... a beautiful creature flying through the air one moment, and then permanent inanimate stillness the next. The young prince was stunned by this experience and began to question life and its obvious mysteries.

He disobeyed his father's wishes and went out of the palace gates into the streets of the city. He saw a strange mixture of misery and suffering ... poverty, hungry people, sad, tortured faces, desperation and anxiety. He saw starving mothers with tiny babes suckling ... small children, almost naked, squabbling over stale breadcrumbs, merchants wrangling to sell their wares, limbless beggars, some blind and crippled, lepers disfigured with untreated weeping sores. He even saw old age and its pain and disfigurement, torture, punishment and death.

The young royal prince had seen in the span of one day the transience of life from birth through desperate survival to eventual death. He saw such a contrast to his abundant palatial existence, that he vowed to go into the world with nothing but the clothes of a beggar and would not rest until he knew the answers to the mysteries.

He made the extreme choice of becoming an ascetic. He began a journey of complete denial of self ... physically and emotionally. He starved himself, only eating the smallest amount of grain. He denied himself comfort, he had no clothes other than a loin cloth, no roof over his head. He denied himself love, family and company, having left his beautiful wife Yashodhara at the palace to raise their child without a father. He spent his time trying even to deny his physical body – not even bathing – in order to reach the consciousness he sought where the answers would be revealed.

One day as he sat by the river, a young merchant boy struggling with a heavy basket of fruits came along the river bank on his way to market. Buddha watched him trip over a stone, his basket falling and spilling its precious contents into the fast flowing waters. Instinctively Buddha struggled with his incredibly weak body to help the boy recover the produce, and having succeeded the boy was very grateful and gave the prince a piece of his fruit. It was then Buddha began to realise that he had gone too far (his pendulum had swung from one extreme in life, to the other).

In the process of helping the young boy, he had bathed his body in water, drank deeply of the water, felt the warmth of another human being, and eaten a piece of fruit and tasted its sweetness.

Life had shown him that the way of the ascetic was not for him ... that he would now travel on his journey through life on the middle path. He could see that nothing could be achieved if we neglected physical and emotional needs, any more than if we overindulge ourselves. He realised that no real benefit could come to mankind by a life of total isolation, any more than a situation where there was never an opportunity for solitude.

The Buddha had come face to face with the amazing truth that life continually changes – like a constant flowing river on its journey to the ocean. The tiny babe becomes the child, the child becomes the adult, the adult becomes old, and death greets everyone without exception.

So it followed that if the physical body would undergo such incredible changes, so the mind and the attitudes would also have the possibility of changing. No situations or circumstances would remain the same forever ... no relationship could endure indefinitely ... everything tangible or intangible must change. (Fascinating here to consider when you look down a busy city street that one hundred years from this moment not one of those people will be here.)

The concept of transience can be quite scary at first because we find ourselves with a huge number of attachments to life. This is where the trust we discover through yoga can be most helpful, because we can also see that difficult and painful situations move on too.

The concept of reincarnation and rebirth can also help us to have a much larger picture when it comes to transience. The theory is that with each lifetime we move on, and even though we need to let go of the past, there is always a new beginning. It is a continual never ending cycle – like the seasons ... spring, summer, autumn, winter ... birth, life, death ... again and again and again.

The bare tree of winter holds the secret of life
Hidden beneath the grey stillness of its trunk
Within the bareness of its limbs ...
Hidden deep within itself is the living spirit
The secret of all creation ... resting, just resting
Dormant to us mere mortals
But alive ... so alive!

When the snows have melted
And the gentle warmth of spring touches the slumbering souls
Held protected in the heart of a tree ...
The stirring starts ... and the whole becomes divided
Hundreds of tiny souls, each with a thirst for life ...
again ...
Another chance for expression
Another chance for progression!
Nature consents and like a "reveille" sounding out the
awakening of a new day ...
Tiny green leaves burst forth ... fresh and crisp
The jewelled tree sings with life once more!

The dancing days of spring pass by too soon ...
And the hot summer sun scorches, scars
A choking thirst for moisture is felt, and sometimes quenched
As leaves grow with maturity, and darken with experience ...
Having suffered, having thrilled
Knowing heat, knowing gale, knowing dryness,
knowing "snail" ...
But feeling the tender touch of God in the coolness
of summer rain
And knowing His peace exists deep within ...
Within the tree itself, within the roots, within the earth.

*The greenness fades and the winds of autumn become
strong and cold
But the sun still shines
And the fight for life begins to mellow
As acceptance fills each leaf with a constant
longing for the soul
Its truest beauty shines forth with brilliant splendour ...
Colours, colours, a vision of brightness
A mass of golds, of reds, of tans
A display of joy ... wisdom ... liberation ...
SAMADHI! ... Bliss
And the world glows with colours that warm the coldest heart
The sun rejoices as its rays sing and dance between the leaves.*

*Coldness ... frosty stillness ... the leaves have
fallen to the earth
Their dance choreographed by the breeze,
the blustering gale, or simply the atmosphere ...
The leaves have fallen, each to dissolve and melt into the earth
To be cradled by the mother earth, to become one with that
nurturing spirit
To feed the tree with new life
To begin again, as the secret circle of life
revolves, revolves ... revolves!*

For people of a Christian or Jewish heritage it is sometimes difficult to understand the "pagan" belief systems of more than one god. The one god is seemingly portrayed as a loving, caring, father figure, but at the same time is to be feared as if He constantly sits in judgement over us so-called disobedient sinners.

However in Hinduism it is a little different. There are six main gods and goddesses worshipped in the temples. Each of these deities represents part of the never ending cycle of birth, life, death. They are so closely linked to the psyche of man you can see them as expressions of your own being or your own needs.

Each god in the male sense has his female consort (just like the love interest of Ida and Pingala). So the balance of the opposites is achieved and the worshipper has a choice depending on their own individual needs.

Brahma is the god of creation, of birth, of new beginnings and his consort is the Goddess Parvati. Brahma as the male component creates by planting the seed, but nothing further can develop unless Parvati is there supplying the fertile ground for conception to occur. To take it into ourselves, Brahma could possibly be explained as the inspiration behind a creative idea, but Parvati is that part of us that manifests the idea into reality.

Vishnu is the Hindu deity of preservation and nurturing. His consort is the Goddess Laksmi. Vishnu, as the masculine aspect, supplies the earth and all its creatures with the necessary ingredients to sustain life ... sunlight, rain, air – whilst Laksmi, the feminine energy, shows us the subtle ingredients of nurturing, love, care, understanding, etc. Vishnu within us can show us how to make a living, to buy the necessary ingredients we need to maintain a certain quality of life – while Laksmi shows us how to nurture, appreciate and even pamper ourselves as well as our loved ones.

In the worship of Vishnu and/or Laksmi we discover the sacredness of life and find the courage to protect it, defend it, save it, rescue it, heal it. Visiting the temple of our own spirit through yoga awareness, we learn more and more to LIVE THAT LIFE.

Siva is the god of destruction and yet transformation. Maybe that is why he is depicted as such an evil image to devotees. His consort is the Goddess Kali, and maybe these two are the most difficult forces to embrace. Siva destroys that which is old, decayed, or even just had its time. Kali helps us to see, in what seems ruthless disposal, cutting down, or actual physical death, how there is a natural need in life to make way for new beginnings, new life.

Siva is that part of our psyche which recognises the need to destroy many aspects of our old thinking. We can all relate in a physical sense as we sometimes need to be almost ruthless in disposing of the "junk" that builds up in our lives. Once gone, out of the way, we have a clean basis to begin again.

The Kali side of our being gives us a sense of clarity, discernment, and the common sense needed in making almost cut-throat decisions to change things. While we are hanging on to all the debris, we are not making progress because the debris eats up our energy, our Prana. (A good test is to look in your wardrobe . . . you will probably see many clothes you haven't worn for years. The simple truth is that if anything is not used it is not loved . . . it drains your Prana, rather than boosting it.)

Connecting with Siva and Kali is a positive step in destroying ignorance. Their strength encourages us to "fire up" and dispose of unused matter or attitudes in the right way. Nature shows us how it is done frequently with bushfires, floods, cyclones, earthquakes, even disease . . . such is the power of destruction.

For us sensitive human beings it is difficult to understand, but without death we have no space for new life to begin. Even in the delicate area of relationships, Siva and Kali show us, no matter how painfully, the importance of detachment at the right time.

However we must also understand that wonderful old things can be given brand new life once Prana (vital energy) is poured into them. Take for example an antique car or piece of furniture, lovingly restored to immaculate condition and treasured by its owner. The alternative is for such items to be ignored, neglected and become scrap.

Of course the same magic applies to human relationships. Nothing is to say that they too cannot be replenished with loving attention and reborn so to speak. Prana is the vital spark to renewal.

To embrace the concept of the six deities, you look into your mind and heart to see that each is part of your psyche. We are on the way to understanding that each individual soul has their own journey through the natural processes of creation, preservation and destruction. The fact of the matter is that not one of us escapes from the cycle of birth, life, death. The truth is sometimes scary, isn't it?

THE "CHRIST" CONNECTION

Most of us in western culture are familiar with the basis of Christianity through the life of Christ as depicted in the first four books of the New Testament of the Bible. Each book was, we are told, written by a devoted disciple of Jesus quite some years after His death on the cross.

The birth, the life, and the death of Christ had such a profound effect on the planet that an incredibly powerful religion was born some 2,000 years ago ... a religion with a basis of love and light, but with an incredible hold over the people by instilling a fear of God, a sense of guilt and shame, as well as destructive self-righteousness. We would all agree that much hypocrisy, cruelty and persecution has occurred down through the ages, all in the name of Christianity, which was the furthest thing from the teachings of Christ.

Consider the man Jesus and everything He stood for, and one sees a self-realised being of light and love, at one with His own divinity which He called God, the Father. He was obviously so in tune with the universe and His own pranic potential that He had the power to transform consciousness, change situations, heal the sick, and the crippled, and even restore life after death.

But you may be asking, "What has yoga to do with Christ?" "What has Christ to do with yoga?"

Let's begin with the Christmas story ... the celebration of Jesus' birth. It is written in the four separate versions that the Christ child was born in a stable in Bethlehem to Mary and Joseph, who was a humble carpenter. There was at the time a particularly bright star overhead, and the beautiful story tells of how shepherds came to pay homage to the newborn babe guided by the star.

Quite amazingly there also came three wise men from the Far East bearing gifts of gold, frankincense and myrrh. They were said to have travelled for many moons (months) and arrived on camels having travelled across vast desert plains. Where could these wise men have come from exactly? How could they have known of such an event? And even more importantly from a human viewpoint, how could they have been bothered making such an amazingly difficult journey? Who were they?

Is there the slightest possibility that these "kings" came from India or Tibet? Could they have been masters of the ancient yoga, so in touch with their higher intuitive minds that they "knew" that this was no "ordinary" birth? Consider the knowledge of the stars that was needed to embark on such a pilgrimage, and trust in the "light" of one special star?

The nativity scene is a feast of archetypes. We can see aspects of ourselves in all the characters.

Mary, the mother ... the feminine side of our being, nurturing, understanding, gentle, compassionate (symbolically the energy of the Nadi, Ida ... the Goddess within).

Joseph, the father ... the masculine aspect of self, protective, responsible, assertive, courageous (maybe the energy of the Nadi, Pingala ... the God within).

The Christ child ... the magical new life that is born when there is union (oneness, yoga) between the mother and the father (the result of loving the whole self ... holiness!). The recognition of the child within helps us to acknowledge how in terms of the universe we are each one of us but a tiny child ... naive, pure in consciousness, open and receptive to new life and new beginnings.

The shepherds represent true humility, which comes naturally from a connection with the heart centre (Anahata Chakra). Following the instincts of the heart means to overcome the resistances of pride and arrogance, awakening true humility which recognises and "bows down in gratitude" to the sacredness of life.

The wise men from the East ... a reflection of that potential of our higher intuitive mind ... that through contemplation, meditation, and self-study, we slowly awaken the magical and creative recesses of our mind (through Ajna Chakra). The picture suggests that we can become more and more aware of that which "we know", and trust completely in that inner knowledge, direction and purpose.

The star ... the absolute symbol of divine spirit, the thread that united all the characters, bringing them to the one place, at the one time ... the ultimate oneness we seek in the transformation of the yoga, when body, mind, heart, unite in spirit.

In the short three years of Christ's mission on earth, He spoke in simple parables or stories as if speaking to children.

It was written that He said ...

"As ye sow, so shall ye reap."
(Yoga interpretation of the teaching of Karma ... cause and effect)

"Love one another."
(An important emphasis on right relationship ... to seek to see the divine love in each other as well as self.)

"In my father's house there are many mansions."
(Yoga interpretation of eternal consciousness containing many incarnations ... or lifetimes.)

"Be still, and know that I am God."
(Emphasises the importance of moments of absolute stillness to become increasingly aware of divine self/spirit ... the yogis would say "I am that".)

"Suffer the little children ... forbid them not."
(Open up to new life, new beginnings, new attitudes, new ideas.)

"Hide not your light under a bushel."
(Let everyone see your true nature, and be true to yourself.)

"Forgive them ... they know not what they do."
(Forgive the faults you see so clearly in others, as the yoga teaches that those faults are aspects of our own being. Beyond all else we need to learn how to forgive ourselves.)

"Let he amongst you who has not sinned throw the first stone."
(Live as best one can without judgement and develop understanding.)

"Don't cast your pearls before the swine."
(As you gain wisdom, be discerning as to whom you share your insights ... for they are the precious jewels of the heart and the mind.)

"The kingdom of heaven is within."
(The simple suggestion that there is only one place to seek the answers ... meditate on the inner space.)

Christ's life was filled with amazing relationships ... people (archetypes) with whom we can so easily relate. Amongst his followers was a prostitute, a publican, simple fishermen, two young women (one who was always seeming to feed the hungry groups whilst the other sat listening at the feet of the master), rich men, poor men, holy men, ascetics ... the list goes on. His life reveals to us His ability to teach and practise the observances and restraints of yoga ... non-violence, honesty, truthfulness, sexual restraint, detachment, cleanliness, contentment, austerity, self-study, and surrender to divine spirit.

Obviously Jesus was a most compassionate human being. It was reported in the Bible that He was so touched by the suffering of those around Him that He began to heal the people, after which He would say "go, and sin no more", almost inferring that it was our own misguided attitudes that had caused the problem in the first place.

He was also quoted as saying to an arrogant man "physician, heal thyself" ... perhaps indicating that through true transformation of attitude we can greatly bring about the healing of our minds and body. Maybe the faith Christ spoke of, is the absolute belief in ourselves.

Jesus healed the sick, the crippled, the blind. He was reported to have brought Lazarus back from the dead. The people adored and idolised Him and made Him more than their teacher (guru) ... they made Him, their God.

The authorities of the time, the high priests and the political leaders no doubt felt extremely threatened and feared the consequence of public uprising. They had no option but to remove the cause of such unnatural adoration and power ... and it was written that none of them was really prepared to take on the full responsibility of what to do with Him.

So in the manner of the day, this innocent but truly enlightened one was betrayed, publicly condemned, tortured, and suffered the dreadful death by crucifixion. As the Roman soldiers nailed Him to the cross, they placed a sign above His head, reading "The King of the Jews".

The body of Christ was said to have been placed in a tomb ... a cave sealed with a rock ... and yet three days after the crucifixion the tomb was visited and the rock had been pushed aside, and there was no body inside.

It was written that He then appeared to Mary Magdalene (who was obviously especially dear to Him) as she walked in a garden. He appeared before His disciples who were gathered together in meeting. He was then recognised by two men on the road to Emmaeus.

It could be comforting to imagine that despite the wondrous theories of most theologians, maybe there was a possibility that

Jesus, the Christ, actually healed Himself, and embarked upon a long journey eastwards ... perhaps, and it is pure speculation, to spend the remaining years of His life in safe seclusion in India and Tibet ... the homeland of the three wise men.

The Serpent

THE SERPENT POWER

The yogis called the powerful energy which we regard as sexual energy, Kundalini. They described it as the serpent power ... a "serpent" coiled at the base of the spine in the earth centre (Mooladhara). It was suggested that after appropriate stimulation, Kundalini would begin to "wake up" and rise as a sensation of uplifted consciousness through the channel of the spine (Sushumna).

On the upwards journey, the Kundalini is said to awaken various Chakras on the way, and on reaching its "full height" at the top of the head would bring about perfect bliss, absolute ecstasy (Samadhi) which we ordinary human beings could identify with "sexual orgasm".

So we begin to realise that sexual energy and spiritual energy are one of the same sacred energy. Yet, somehow we have, through our attitude to life, put them in very separate categories. Again it is how we use our mind and our imagination that affects this incredible energy. Sex can be as far removed from spirituality as one likes. The pompous, pious Victorian attitude was that sex was only acceptable in a married state of love – apart from that it was something "of the devil", a giving into the temptation of lust and desire, and certainly not acceptable to God. Yet could one truly say that all marriages were "made in heaven"?

The masters of the yoga discovered that this Kundalini energy would rise upwards not just in sexual union but as the result of the consciousness slowly transforming in meditation. This transmutation could eventually produce an ecstatic and yet peaceful state of bliss the yogis called Samadhi. This experience of LOVE was so overwhelming and all embracing that one was "IN LOVE" with the entire universe. Such experience on a regular basis was found to awaken amazing creative potential as if the Kundalini had released dormant talent and inspiration.

Living in a time where very young adolescents experiment with sex so freely, it could be worthwhile encouraging yoga and meditation into the school curriculum as a means of tapping the serpent power (Kundalini) and harnessing its vital creative energy. Such practices could help to overcome immature frustrations and give young people clear directions and a passionate approach to more worthwhile and fulfilling activities.

After sexual orgasm one feels that same sense of peace and love of course, but it seems to have only a limited affect on the psyche, whereas the meditational experience actually transforms the practitioner. The message, of course, is balance ... the middle path as Buddha called it. Too much Samadhi experience in meditation could cause one to become a recluse, an ascetic, retreating from the world. On the other hand, too much sex could cause one to become greedy, with an insatiable appetite for sexual gratification, which when taken to extremes could become so out of control that perverse and deviant behaviour follows, where the sexual partner becomes a victim and not a lover.

The practice of the yoga is the greatest aid to keeping the scales beautifully balanced ... hence discovering a healthy, holy, experience of ever-increasing selfless LOVE. Love insures that there is never any space at all for enforcing power over others, or invasion into another's space. It is suggested that personal fulfilment can be discovered through the universal law of giving generously of self ... just as one opens unconditionally to receive.

The ancient Tantra yoga, sometimes referred to as the yoga of sexual union, suggests that in making love wonderful experiences of bliss can be attained by regarding your lover as truly divine. In other words to make love to your man as if he was a God ... to make love to your woman as if she was a Goddess ... to see the God/Goddess within your lover.

The yogis knew that this powerful Kundalini was the most sacred energy, and not something we could take for granted. It is the absolute basis of our connection with spirit ... our very physical existence is dependent on its magic. Opposites attract ... man and woman unite ... the Kundalini rises and a new life is conceived. We begin to see that we are the precious instruments in the never ending cycle of life.

There is no denying that sexual oneness is a spiritual experience. Once we understand the sacredness of that amazing energy which can be used sexually, creatively and/or spiritually, we are discovering that we are truly filled with divine magic.

RELATIONSHIP AND SOLITUDE

In terms of Karma and reincarnation, relationships are most certainly wonderful opportunities to balance the scales from previous lifetimes ... In other words to work through problems that exist between us, and attend to any unfinished business left over from "last time" together.

You can be sure that you are in relationship at this time, in this place, because you are linked by Karma ... and that concept embraces not just a few, but the multitudes ... the intimate "family" right through to the global "family". Indifference to another would indicate that there is no karmic "sorting out" necessary between you ... but if you find yourself reacting to another's actions or words, feeling hurt or angry, it is obvious there is still a karmic debt to be paid between you.

Without relationship, loving or unpleasant, beautiful or trying, we would never glimpse true images of ourselves through the magical mirror that is another human being. Whether we like it or not, the things that annoy us most in the actions and attitudes of others are undoubtedly the traits we dislike so much about ourselves. In philophonetic psychology, we can actually be shown the truth of this.

On a more positive note, relationships also show us the love, the compassion, the joy in others. This appreciation is also a clear mirror of our very own "goodness". The more evolved each one of us becomes, the easier it is to see the divine spark that glows in every human being. Relationships are the precious links that unite us all in the never ending cycle of spirit.

Solitude on the other hand is so necessary to enable us to commune with that divine spark that is truly glistening in our own heart and mind. Such "aloneness" (not to be confused with loneliness) gives us the opportunity to practise the yoga, to release conflict through prayer, to meditate and be with stillness, to delight in the wondrous beauty of nature, be it the earth or the sky.

As life progresses many gateways open and yet close to us. In looking back through the years one sees that we have made many choices in life which have taken us along many different pathways The result of choice making (good or bad) has meant that some relationships have broken down and even disappeared. (In the process of "looking at" what has gone before, it is quite a good exercise to establish whether you feel there is still unfinished business or do you feel completely free from past relationships.)

We pass through new gateways and we may find ourselves embarking on brand new grounds of relationship, testing us still further, or making us feel more comfortable with who we truly are. All that is asked of us is to allow for the flow of life, trust and open our hearts to what it brings to us. The timing and the magnetism is always astounding. We are told by the masters of the yoga that there are no mistakes in life, only more lessons to be learned!

As we grow in awareness so solitude becomes increasingly meaningful to connect us with spirit. Through solitude it is easier to make clear choices, have a vision of purpose and direction, learn discretion and discernment, gain sufficient strength to always be true to self, and become receptive to inspiration and creative energy.

Loneliness is something else again ... It comes about when spiritual growth pauses or even stops ... when a person closes up the heart and the mind to further growth experiences, and no longer searches the smorgasbord of possibilities and choice that life constantly offers us.

We recognise this loneliness in the elderly when the spirit is tired and just marking time awaiting death. But unfortunately we often see it in the young who have not been shown how to grasp life in their hands as their natural birthright. In such people there are feelings of unworthiness, a lack of self esteem. They feel that they are not deserving of that which is just waiting for them around the next bend in the road.

Yoga teaches us that our happiness in life is completely up to each one of us and our own attitude towards it. Our happiness is certainly not dependent on the words or actions of any other human beings. Understanding the truth of that, we are in an excellent position to enjoy the spontaneous and unpredictable nature of every relationship, being continually open to learning, and balancing out the experiences bathing in solitude.

The Postures

THE POSTURES, THE BREATHING, THE FEELING

The postures of the yoga are called Asanas and many have been given the names of animals and creatures obviously because the forms emulate not only the shape of the creature, but also the unique attitude involved.

From a physical point of view the Asanas stimulate internal organs and in particular the endocrine glands, therefore balancing hormones.

There are also certain practices called Mudras which involve hand movement and positions, which are not unlike the beautiful gestures of Eastern dancers. Such practices cannot help but centre awareness and transform consciousness bringing incredible feelings of humility, tranquillity, peace and gratitude.

Each Asana has its own choice of counterpose to release tension and ensure balance. You will see the continuing influence of masculine and feminine energies with outward extensions and inward folding.

The breathing practices are called Pranayamas ("Prana" meaning vital life force, and "Yama" meaning 'to control' or 'to direct'). There are many such practices obviously designed to polarise the opposite energies (Pingala ... sun energy ... masculine, and Ida ... moon energy ... feminine) within the body of light, to direct Prana through the Sushumna, to awaken and align the Chakras, and increase concentration skills.

It is the aim of the yogi to combine the chosen Asana with a suitable Mudra, and Pranayama (i.e. awareness of posture, attitude and breath simultaneously).

The wonderful thing is that the yoga is suitable for everyone, all ages, all shapes and sizes, all nationalities, all beliefs, all backgrounds. Its aim is to unite, not divide, to help us discover the universal consciousness which is the source of our being and to which we all belong.

However it is important when considering the practice of yoga to seek out an experienced teacher capable of awakening you to the fine details of each Asana, Pranayama and Mudra. Attention to physical detail with each and every practice is imperative to caring for the body. But the physical posture alone is not yoga. It is only when the mind and heart are fully focussed in the present moment ... be it with breath awareness, attitudinal feeling, sound vibration, or creative visualisation ... that the state of yoga is reached.

And then, even then the masters suggest, we have only just begun the journey towards SPIRIT!

POSTURES OF COURAGE (Masculine)

The more "geometric" Asanas like Trikonasana (Triangle Pose) require dedicated practice to perfect but promise you good physical posture, co-ordination, and an awareness of inner strength and courage to help overcome the fears and anxieties of life.

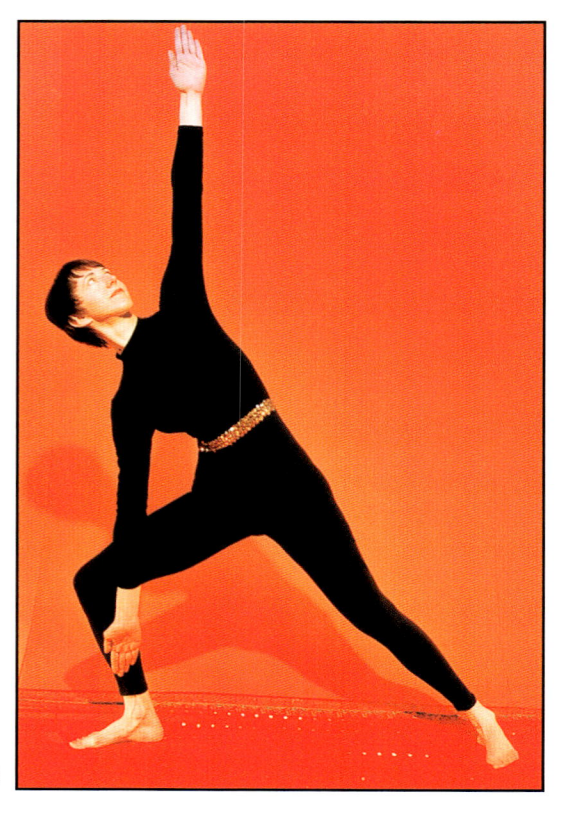

Trikonasana (Triangle Pose)

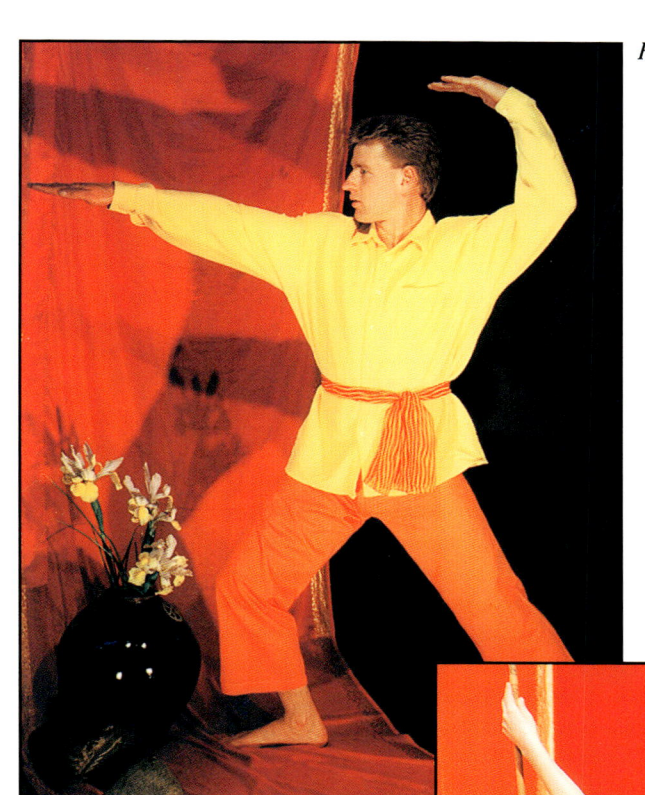

Hero Pose

Ushtrasana Variation (Camel Pose)

POSTURES OF HUMILITY (Feminine)

These Asanas are to do with folding up, maybe like the bud of a flower or in a foetal position ... "to become as a tiny child" and enjoy all that goes with that experience ... the pure delight, the wonder, the naivety, the gratitude, the humility. Also the experience of unfolding can be an absolute joy, like a "new beginning".

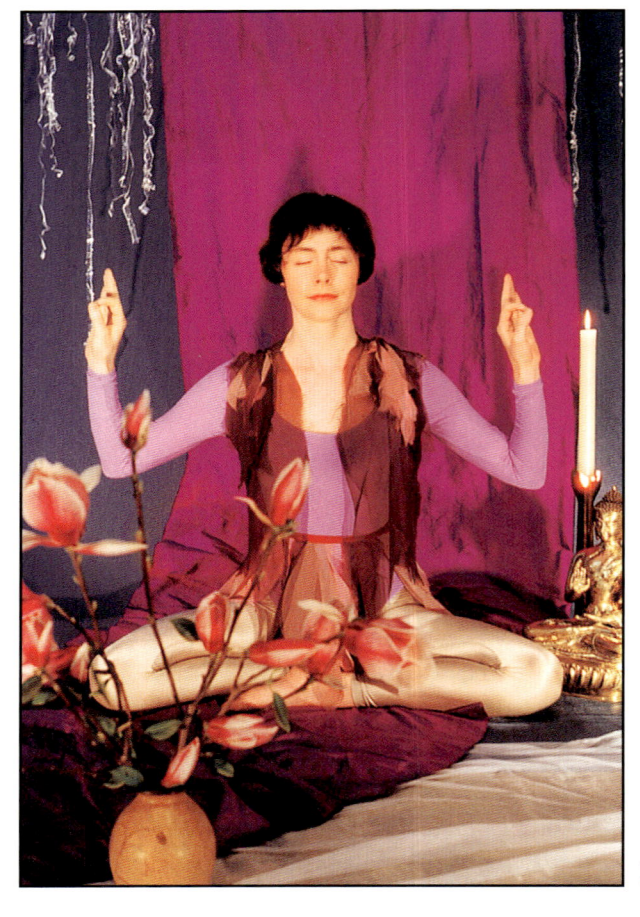

Yoga Mudra (Humility Pose)

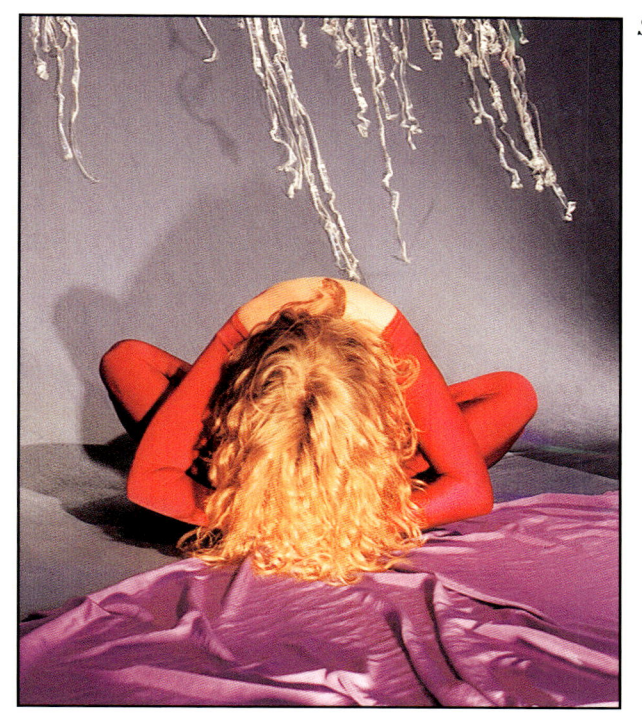

Star Pose

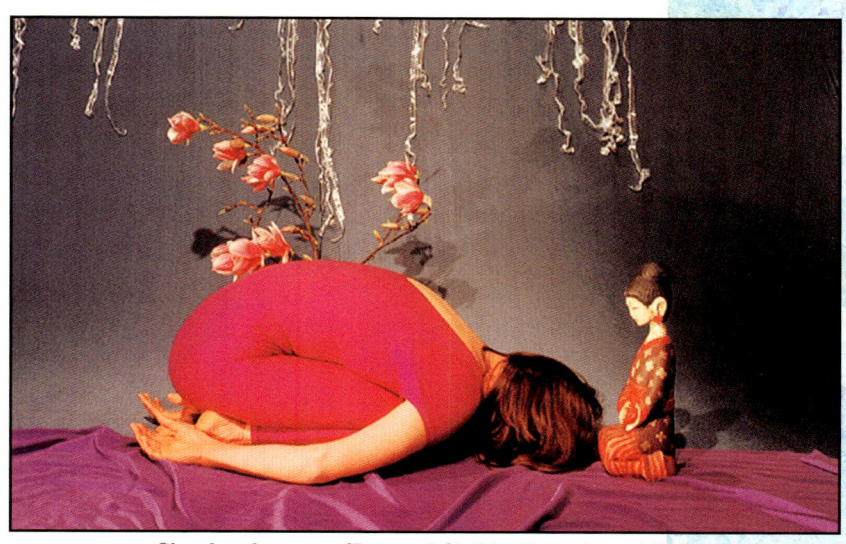

Shashankasana (Pose of Child – foetal position)

POSTURES OF STRENGTH (Masculine)

You will find these postures work on awakening a number of energy centres, but there is a strong focus on the fire centre at the solar plexus. We are looking at not only physical strength, but psychological and spiritual strength. A strength which comes from suppleness and flexibility, not force and struggle.

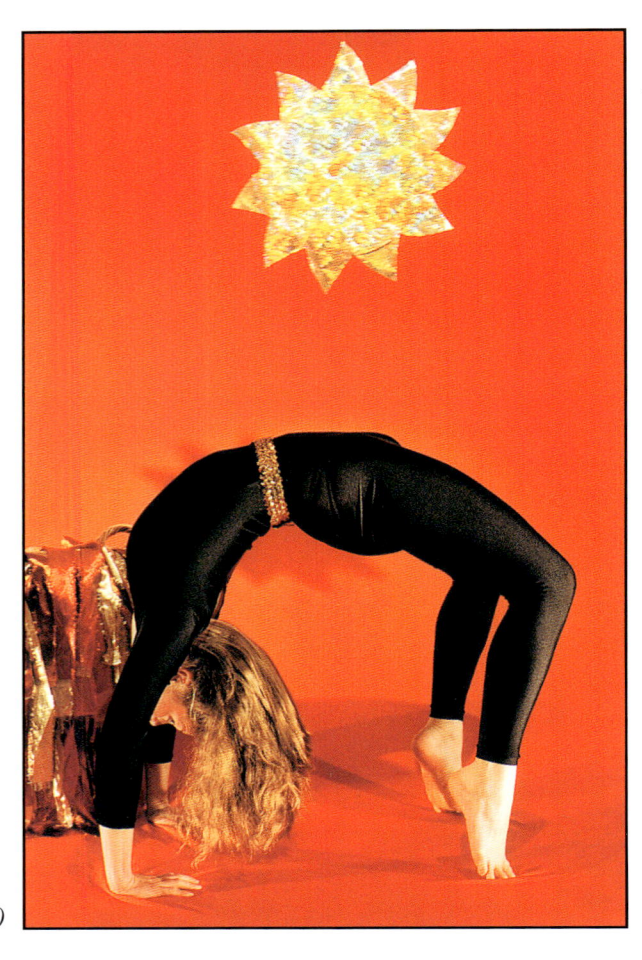

*Chakrasana
(Wheel/Bridge Posture)*

Dhanurasana (Bow Posture)

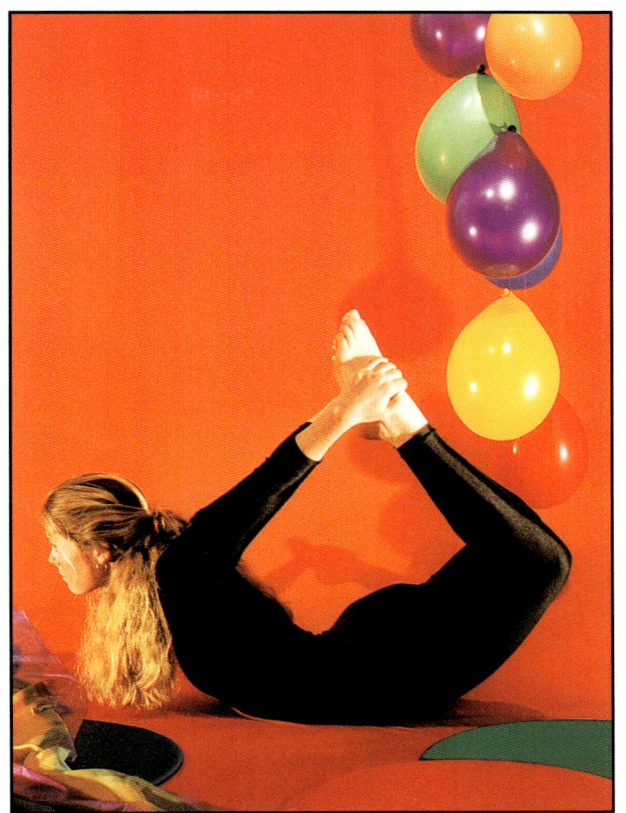

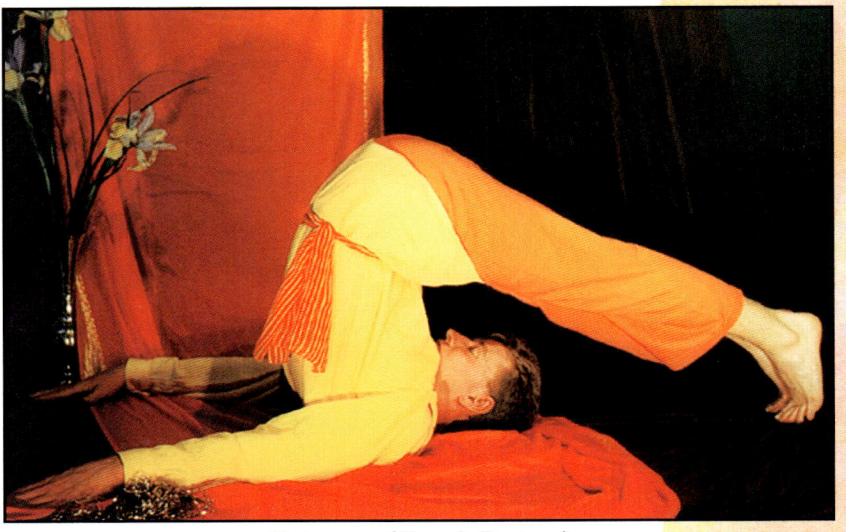

Halasana (Plough Posture)

POSTURES OF TRANQUILLITY (Feminine)

Tranquillity brings about an experience of inner peace, serenity and gentle contentment just "TO BE" in the chosen posture. They are usually Asanas that become your favourites because you feel so comfortable and at ease while the process of centring takes care of itself, and the awareness is pure enchantment.

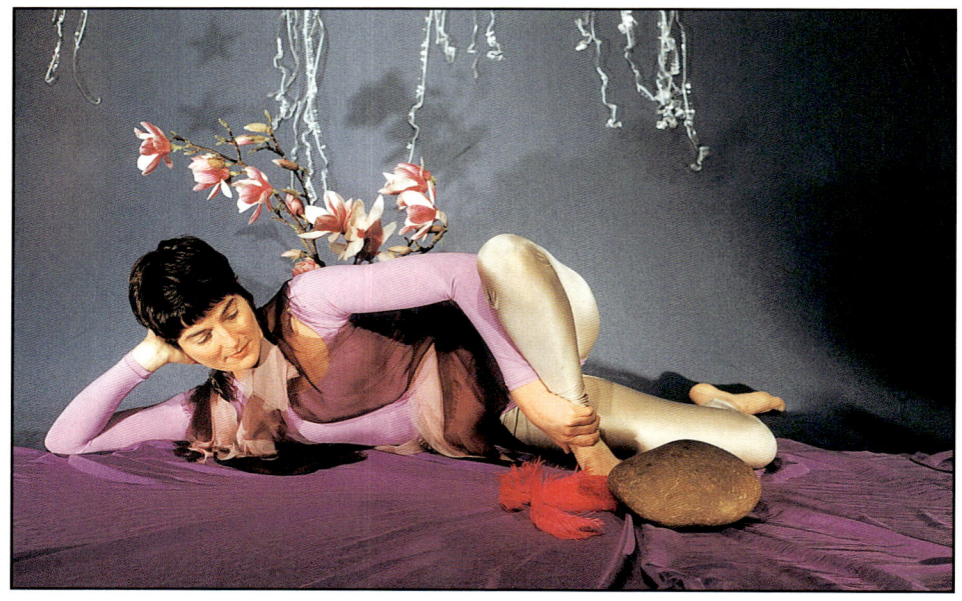

Buddha's Reclining Pose

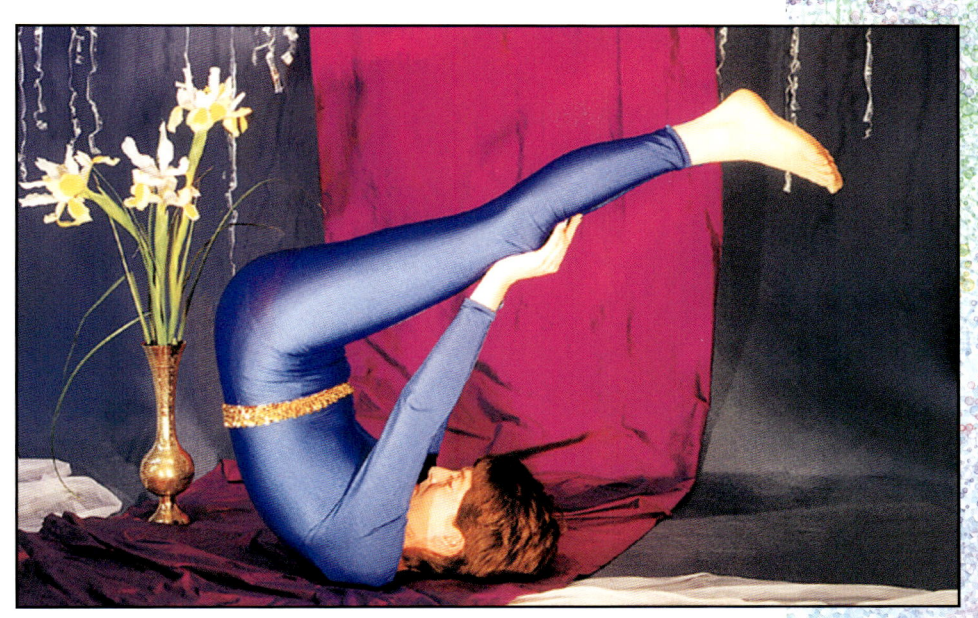

Pose of Tranquillity

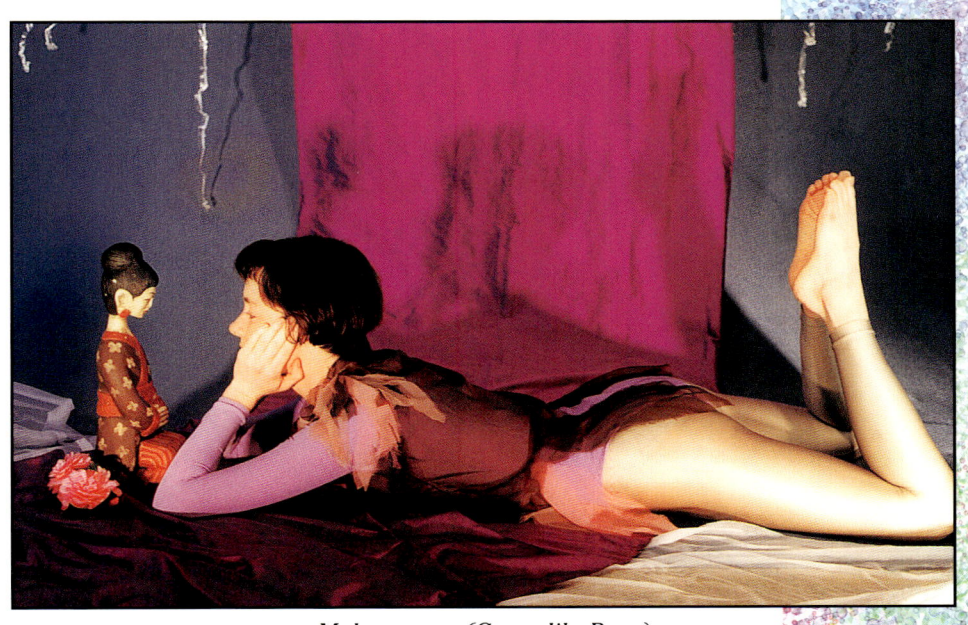

Makarasana (Crocodile Pose)

POSTURES OF CONFIDENCE (Masculine)

These Asanas you will discover emphasise the heart centre by expanding the chest cavity, strengthening the heart and the lungs and increasing breath capacity. Once the heart centre is alive and filled with light, so our self-image improves dramatically giving us the self-esteem and confidence to tackle anything that comes our way.

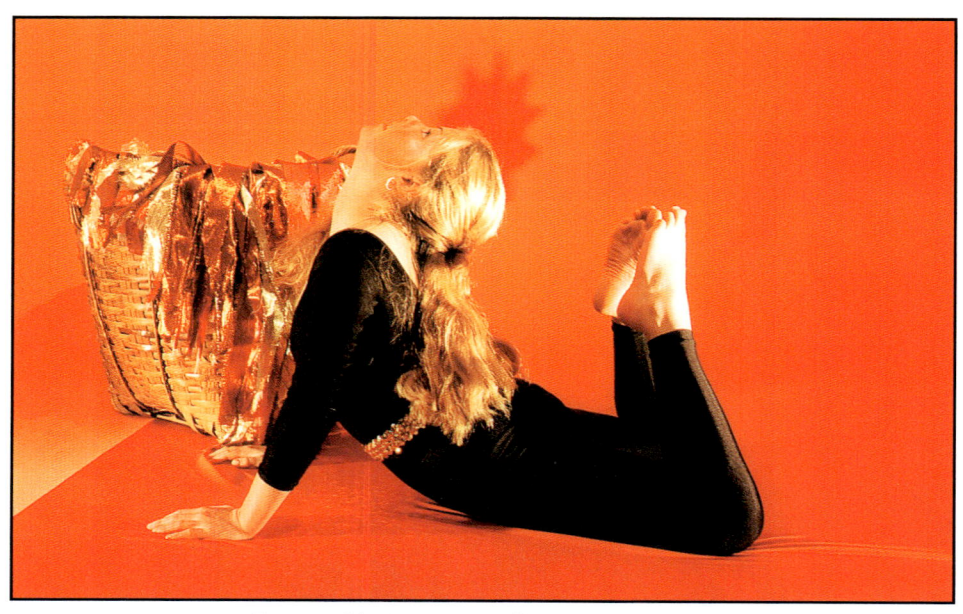

Poorna Bhujangasana (King Cobra Pose)

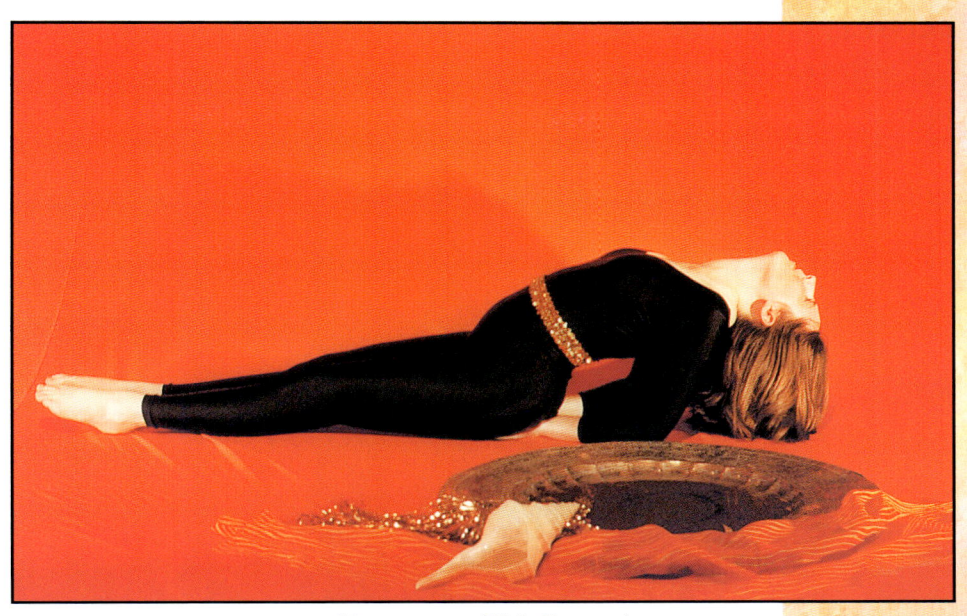

Matsyasana (Fish Posture)

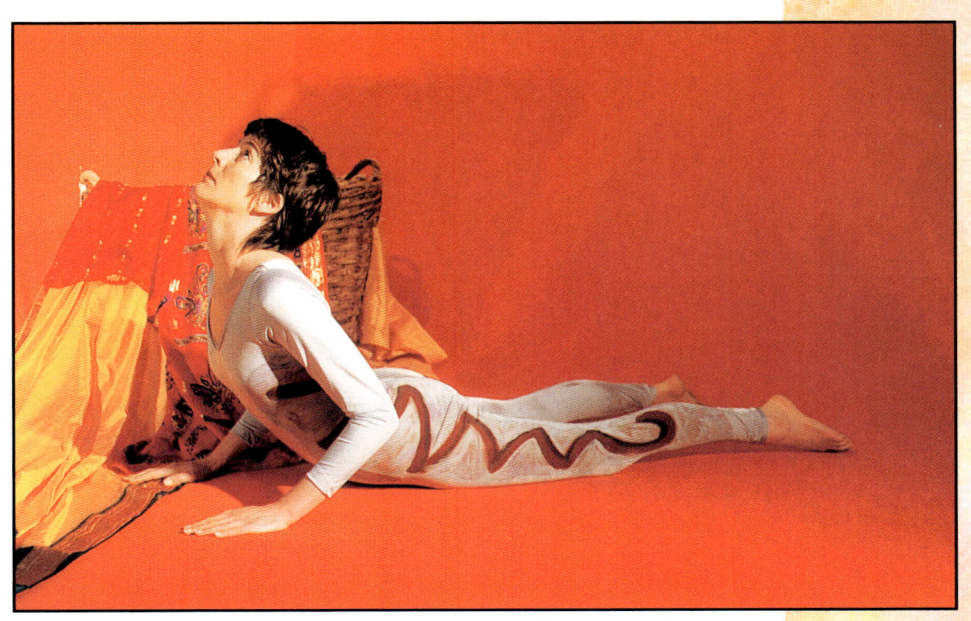

Bhujangasana (Easy Cobra Pose)

POSTURES OF SURRENDER (Feminine)

Surrender means absolute "letting go" and "giving in". The Asanas are forward bending which require a real sense of dissolving all resistances and melting. In most cases the holding of the posture a little allows the necessary time and space for the appropriate "giving in" to take place. The result is patience, understanding and an ever-increasing trust in life.

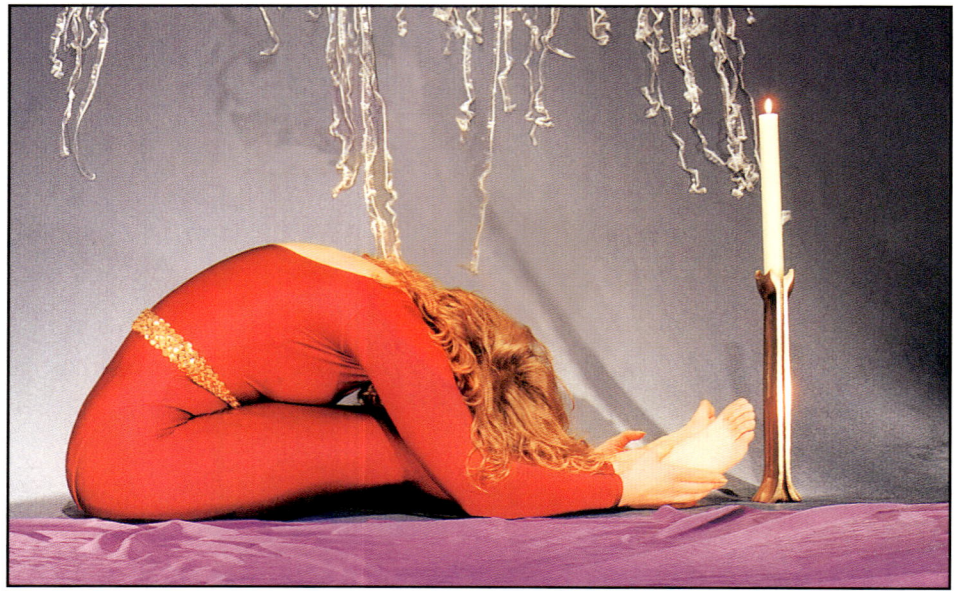

Paschimottanasana (Forward Bend)

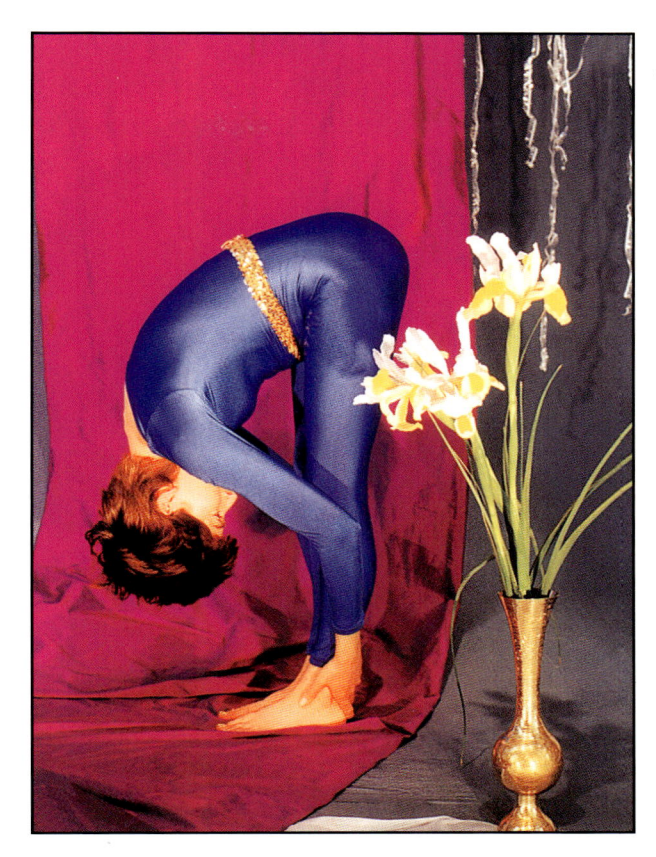

Padahastasana
(Jack Knife Posture)

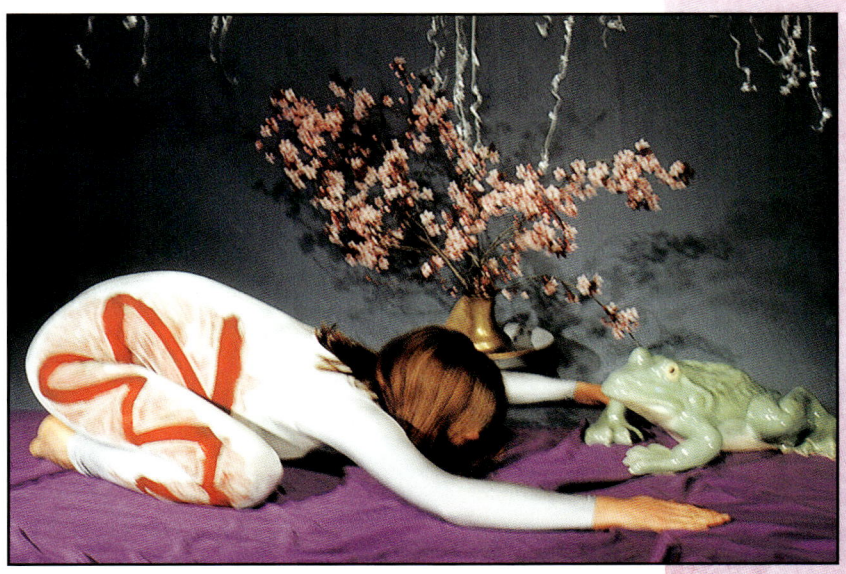

Flat Frog Posture

59

POSTURES OF BALANCE (Masculine)

These Asanas require absolute one-pointed awareness and therefore are a wonderful prerequisite for meditation preparing the mind to be focussed in the present moment. Balancing practices can be helpful to develop powers of concentration.

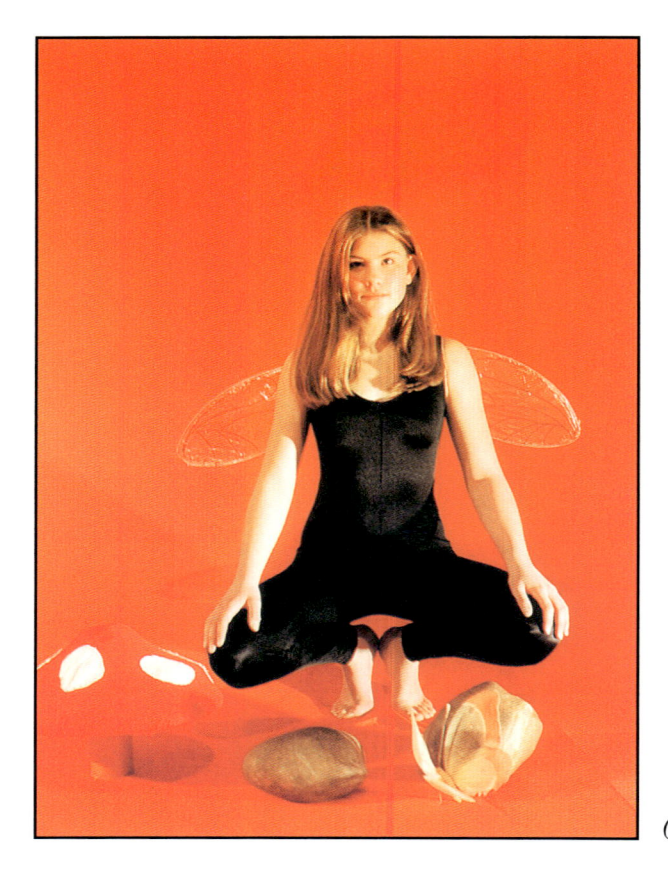

Bakasana
(Bird Perching Pose)

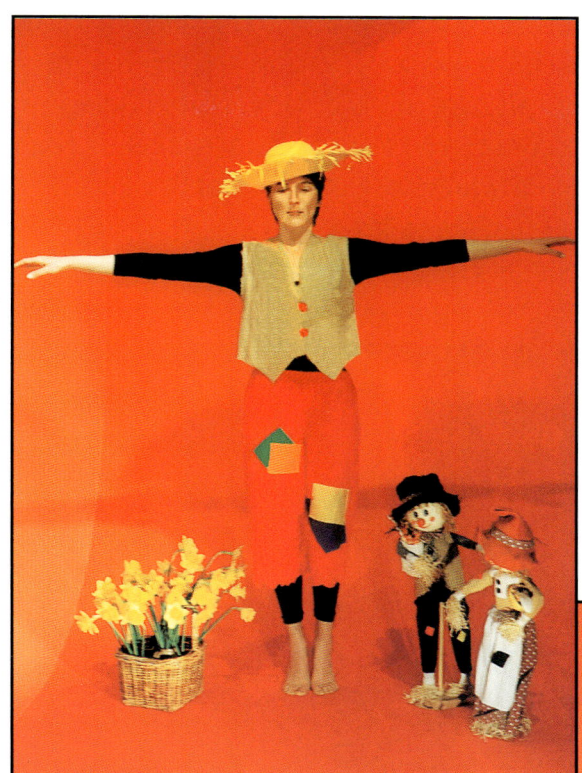

*Tadasana Variation
(Scarecrow Pose)*

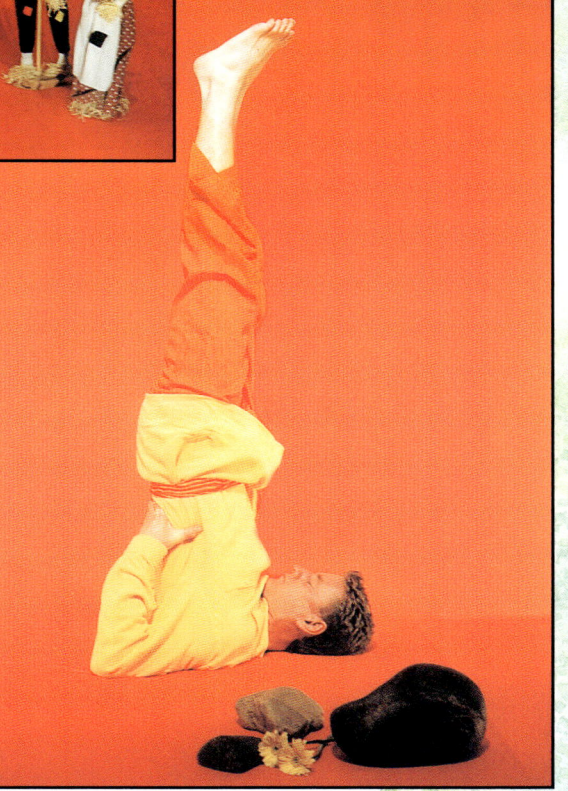

*Sarvangasana
(Candle Pose)*

POSTURES OF GRACE (Feminine)

These are steady Asanas that speak of "sitting up" rather than "sitting down" ... being totally at ease uniting body, mind and spirit. Candle gazing can instill a quiet elegance like a graceful swan drifting upon the surface of still water (the stillness of the mind).

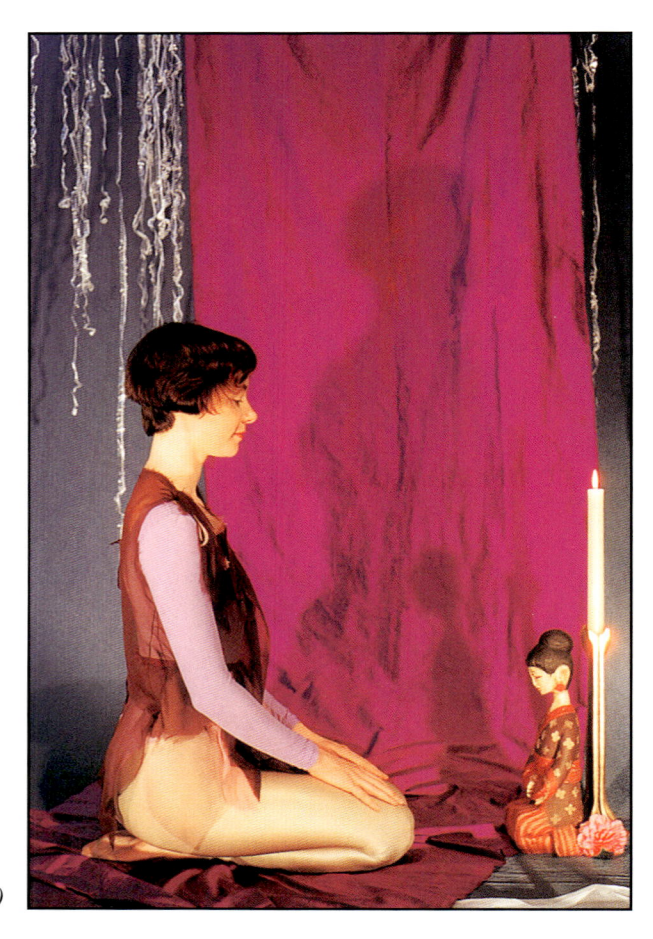

Vajrasana
(Thunderbolt Pose)

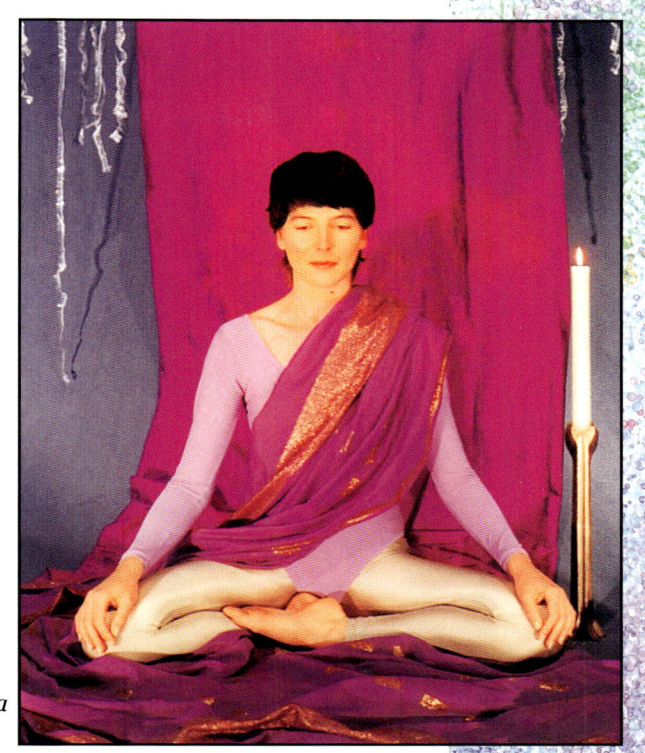

*Siddhasana with Chin Mudra
(Accomplished Pose)*

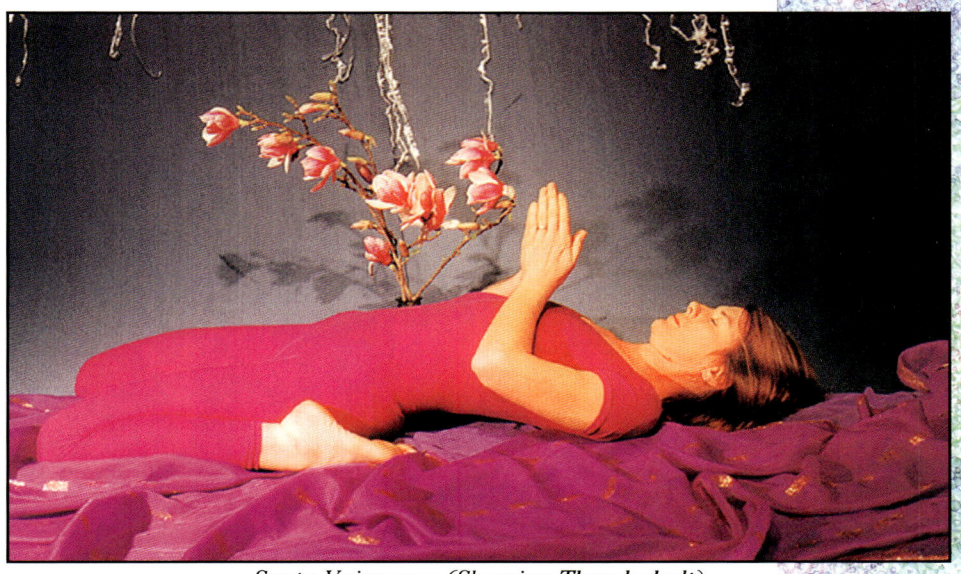

Supta Vajrasana (Sleeping Thunderbolt)

POSTURES OF DIGNITY (Masculine)

The spinal twists of the yoga certainly bring about a feeling of dignity, awakening more and more a sacred respect for human potential and being. The powerful twists work towards a stronger nervous system and increased coping ability.

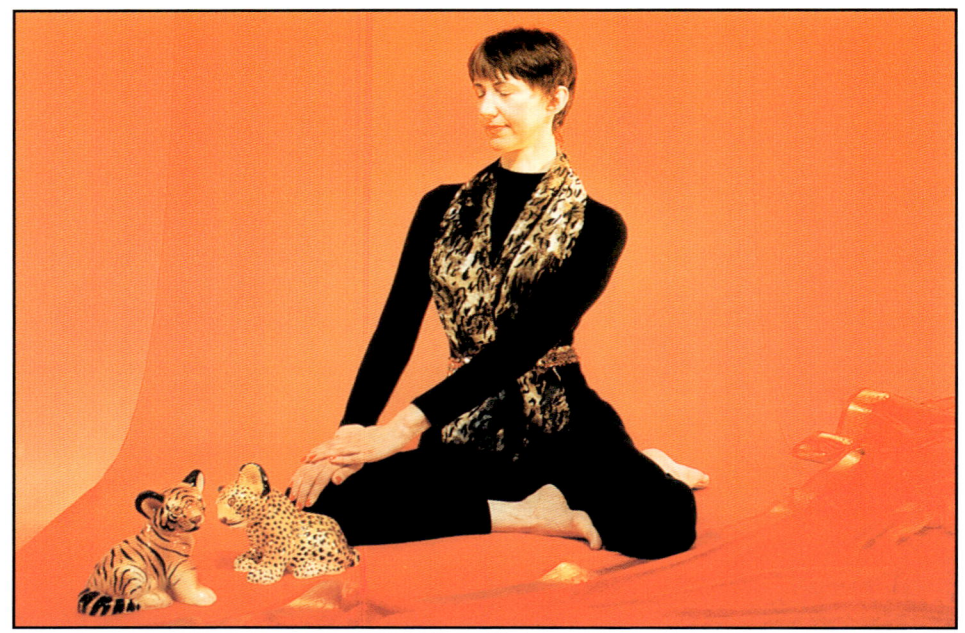

Tiger Sitting

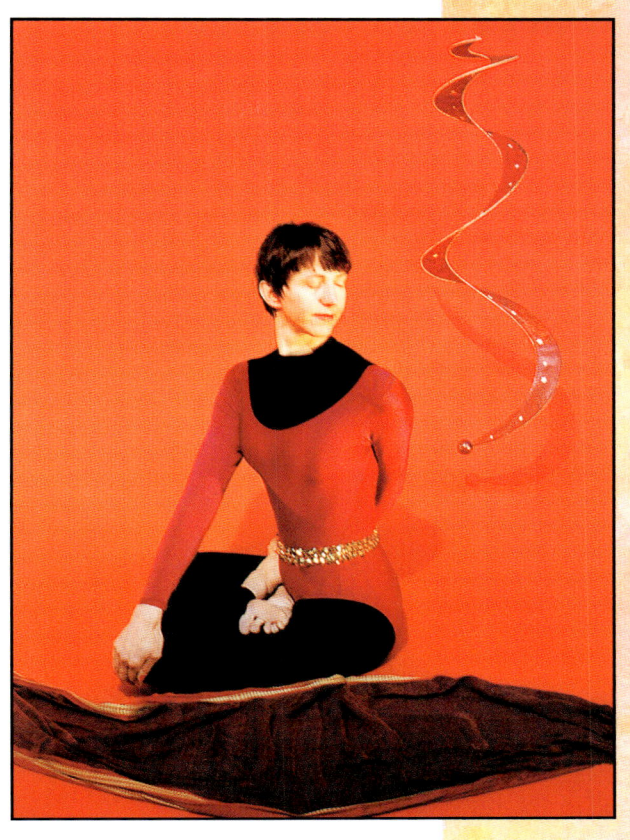

*Matsyendrasana Variations
(Spine Twists)*

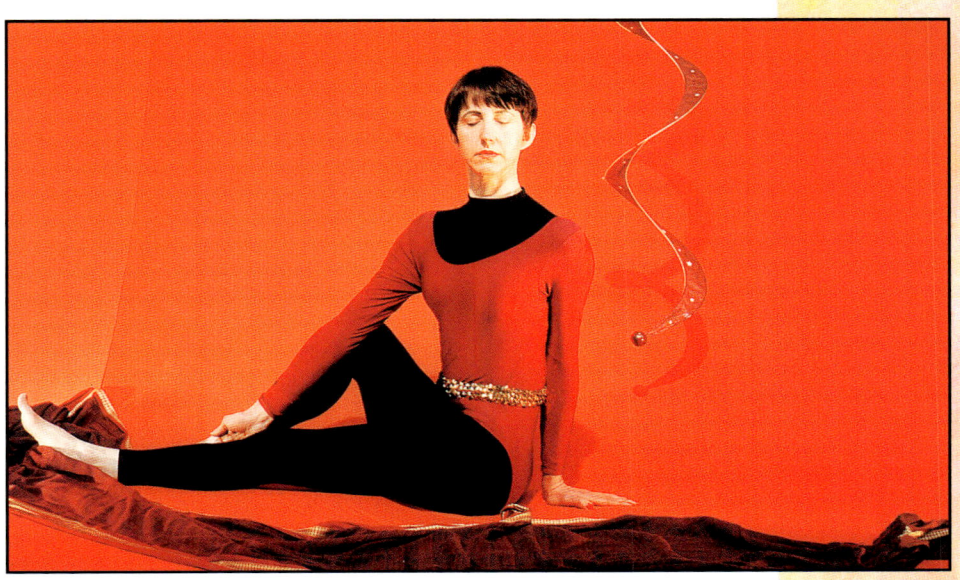

POSTURES OF DIVINITY (Feminine)

These Asanas and/or Mudras invoke divine light (in other words "enlightenment"). The practitioner enjoys a sense of glowing and total well being. The experience is a mixture of joy, delight, purity, perfection, oneness with "what is"! Become THAT LIGHT!

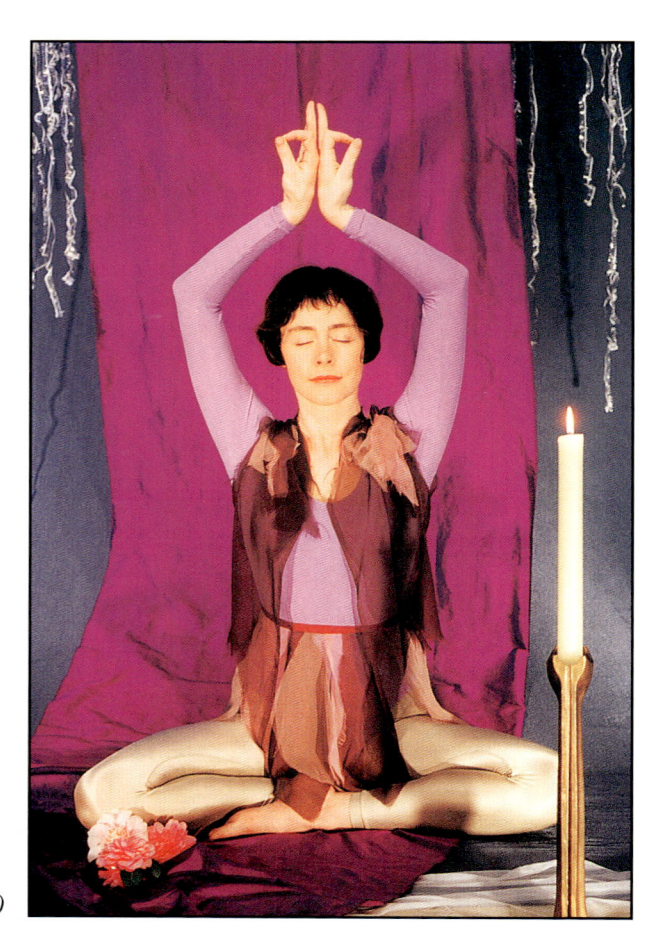

*Siddhasana
(Temple Goddess Mudra)*

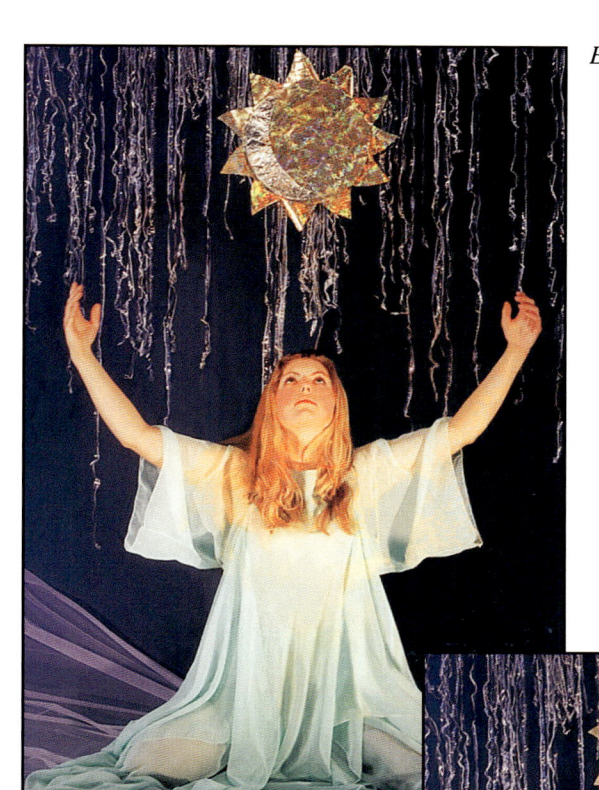

*Bhadrasana with
Prana Mudra*

*Bhadrasana
with Yoga Mudra*

Meditation

MEDITATION PLUS RELAXATION = HEALING

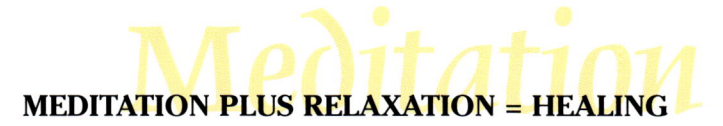

The definition of yoga as stated in the ancient texts of the Yoga Sutras says:

"Yoga is the inhibition of the modifications or fluctuations of the mind."

Many times meditation is confused with attempting to stop the thinking process, when in reality one never stops thinking, but rather embarks on a journey through various yoga practices or techniques in order to enchant the mind and therefore to tame it. In other words yoga brings the thinking process into a central focal point and maintains that focus.

The amazing thing is that wherever the focus of the mind is, there the Prana (life force) is directed. For instance if you are building a boat and that project becomes the centre of your attention, a very large amount of your creative energy will go into that boat, and it would be a pretty close bet that the result would be quite amazing. If, however your interest was only half-hearted, the result would reflect that. So the same theory extends into everything we do in life ... where our main focus is, so is our energy, and there certainly can be a negative side to that.

If, for instance, we have an obsession or an addiction of any kind, that absorbs most of our Prana, the obsession/addiction will undoubtedly grow. If we have a rift in a relationship which creates ill feeling, animosity and hurt, and we focus continually upon that problem, the feeling escalates into bitterness, resentment and/or anger. It is not difficult to see how harmful such things can be to our health.

Relaxation techniques of the yoga (Nidra) are specially designed to refocus the thinking process in positive directions in order to redirect the flow of Prana towards beauty, light, love and joy, so that natural healing can result.

If we can develop our creative visualisation as to imagine bathing the whole being in glorious light, we are actually bathing the physical body in positive healing pranic energy. When we have a particularly weakened part of our body (pain, injury or disease) and we are able to train the mind not to sink into despair, but rather fill the area with beautiful "blue-green" healing colours, we could be contributing very positively to a natural healing process.

When we discuss meditation, most people think of a yogi (like a statue of Buddha) sitting cross-legged in lotus posture with a very straight back, eyes closed, and distant attitude, for hours on end. But even though all of the yoga postures and breathing practices bring us slowly towards the contentment and discipline of such a "sitting", one cannot deny here in the West, that there are a multitude of ways a person can derive certain benefits not unlike meditation ... that is taking into consideration that meditation could be defined as centring awareness to one focal point and maintaining that focus.

Consider why so many men and women enjoy to go fishing. Is it just the catch, or are there those beautiful people who love the connection with soothing water, the quietness, the solitude, the oneness? The same experience of spirit can be felt by consciously aware individuals standing high on a mountain top absorbing the breathtaking scenery, or quietly strolling through a beautiful garden, along a vast deserted beach, sitting beside a quiet lake listening to the lulling, lapping of water against the shore, or simply drinking in the fragrance of a rose.

Some people would suggest that this experience of consciousness shifting could be called "day-dreaming" and yet such inner visions of such experiences are conducive to deep relaxation producing a real sense of well being and wholeness.

It could be suggested that day-dreaming could be a subtle form of meditation, and yet the yogic masters warn against allowing ourselves to drift into sleep or unconsciousness. There is no denying we all need a good balance of rest and sleep in order to rejuvenate the being. In observing new born infants (who have just arrived into the physical world from spirit) and elderly folk (who are drawing closer to uniting with spirit once again) both need so much more sleep, which seems to be a natural transition between earth and spirit.

Meditation, however, is that we may become one with spirit on a regular basis throughout our busy, creative, active day-to-day life. It requires the full attention of an alert, awake mind. A mind that is prepared to seek ...

... the stillness that occurs between each breath

... the silence that is beyond sound

... the empty space that is between each outside thought

Obviously when the mind has been seduced by the constant external stimulation of life, this is not such an easy task, and it certainly requires a huge dedication and commitment. However when the heart has suffered hurt and disillusionment sufficiently in life, there seems to come naturally a deep inner yearning for spirit contact, and that alone might be all that is required as the springboard to transformation. Note that it most possibly has taken many lifetimes of experience to really see and accept the need for looking within oneself for true happiness. Us human beings are noted right through history for being quite resilient for falling into the same hopeless traps again and again.

The yogis suggest that as idealistic as it seems the true nature of mankind is happiness and the responsibility of discovering THAT is our very own. Meditation is possibly an important process along the way to enlightenment, which the masters called Samadhi.

Some teachers of the yoga suggest that when the keen aspirant has practised sufficient postures to feel comfortable in a sitting position for a reasonable time (perhaps 10-20 minutes to begin) constant Mantra repetition is valuable. Mantra is a vibrational sound which has a lulling, relaxing effect on the practitioner. For instance, to a tiny babe the sound of a mother humming a lullaby is soothing. As adults we find such sounds as humming bees, rolling waves, gentle breezes, relaxing. The yogis say that within the lulling sounds of nature is the universal sound "OM" which when verbalised takes on the fullness of three separate sounds ..."A" "U" "M" – creating a wonderful vibration down the spine (Sushumna).

The masters of the yoga, the gurus, were known to give each of their disciples or devotees a personal Mantra (a ceremony called "Mantra Initiation") to silently repeat upon the constant rhythmical movement of their breath throughout their meditation times. Such Mantras have always been considered truly special and sacred, and kept quite secret. More universally used Mantras for example are: Om-So-Ham ... Ham-So ... So-Ham ... Om Shanti ... and these too are extremely powerful and effective.

Certain Pranayamas (breathing techniques) are very useful to calm and centre the mind in preparation to meditation. The alternate nostril breathing (Nadi Shodhan) balances the energies of Ida and Pingala into a central point of consciousness. The warming breath of Ujjayi creates a rich humming sound inside which lulls and comforts. The cooling breath of Sheetkali and Sheetkari awakens the eyebrow centre Ajna to truly focus the mind.

Practices which involve deep concentration on sound (Antar Mouna ... inner silence) from external sound to internal sound, and even beyond, can also be extraordinarily helpful. One discovers even silence has a sound.

Candle gazing (Tratak) is a simple but most effective method of developing creative visualisation skills, which enhance ideas and inspiration.

It is suggested that an aspirant is wise to seek out a good teacher of the yoga in order to learn these practices with loving guidance.

The truly enlightened ones upon our planet have never boasted of countless mind-blowing spiritual experiences of lights and angelic visitations, but each taught constantly the power of LOVE and PEACE ... possibly because in the deepest states of meditation they knew first hand that within their own conscious awareness lay the real possibility of becoming THAT LOVE, THAT PEACE ... simply THAT!

THE DANCE OF THE YOGA

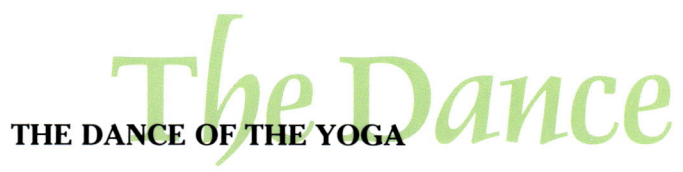

Once we understand how the postures of the yoga awaken certain attitudes because of the centres and elements that are triggered in those postures, we can begin to connect the still forms into a continuous flowing practice ... in other words movement.

For example in the classic yoga of old there is a practice called Surya Namaskara (salutation to the sun) which involves twelve Asanas (postures). The combination of those Asanas continually opens, closes, and extends the body, filling the being with a sense of sunlight which when focussed upon becomes Prana (vital energy). The practitioner cannot help feeling filled to the brim with self-esteem, wonder, appreciation, humility, strength, courage, and delight, all in the one experience. One could call it a prayer in movement. Its continual practice seems to develop the masculine aspects of positivity, stamina, and a sense of achievement.

Down through the ages more and more creative versions of postures connecting into movement developed. Chandra Namaskara (salutation to the moon) ... producing feelings of soft moonlight releasing resistances, visions of silvery moonlight on water, humility but dignity and contentment, solitude and yet oneness.

The elephant series of postures seem to mimic this large creature. Its trunk dipping down into the water and earth ... its amazing strength of charging through the dense jungle, its tusks, and its need to give into its own heaviness.

One begins to realise that there is no limit to where one goes with posture and movement ... in fact it would be absurd to suggest that there are only 84 yoga postures, for the introduction into 84 experiences only plants the seeds for a never ending discovery of multitudes of variations and combinations. Just as we are blessed with amazing talent in every field, be it medicine, technology, art, film, literature, construction, music, drama, so it is with yoga. There is always the possibility for growth and expansion.

Creative dance has its base in yoga awareness. It takes the elements and character of the centres of the body ... i.e. earth, water, fire, air, space and beyond, and instead of being contained in still form allows it to flow in movement. Music or idea becomes the magic choreographer of the dance that evolves.

Music, the language of the universe, is always of one or more elements. For instance, broadly speaking the primitive musics of the indigenous peoples, say, the Australian Aboriginal people, African negroes, Native American Indians, with such percussion instruments as drums, sticks, rocks, and wonderful inspiring "heart" instruments like the didjeridoo and the rain maker, awaken the Earth Chakra at the base of the spine. The dance it brings about is of the pelvic floor, with feet firm against the earth ... stomping, thumping, etc.

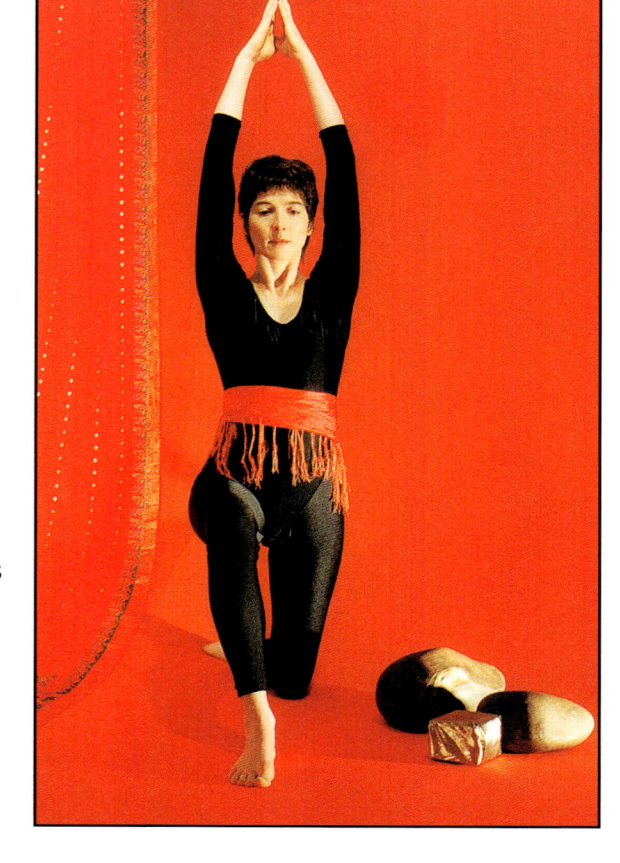

THE ELEPHANT involves a series of linking postures depicting the trunk, the ears, and the tusks ... aspiration, strength and surrender to heaviness.

75

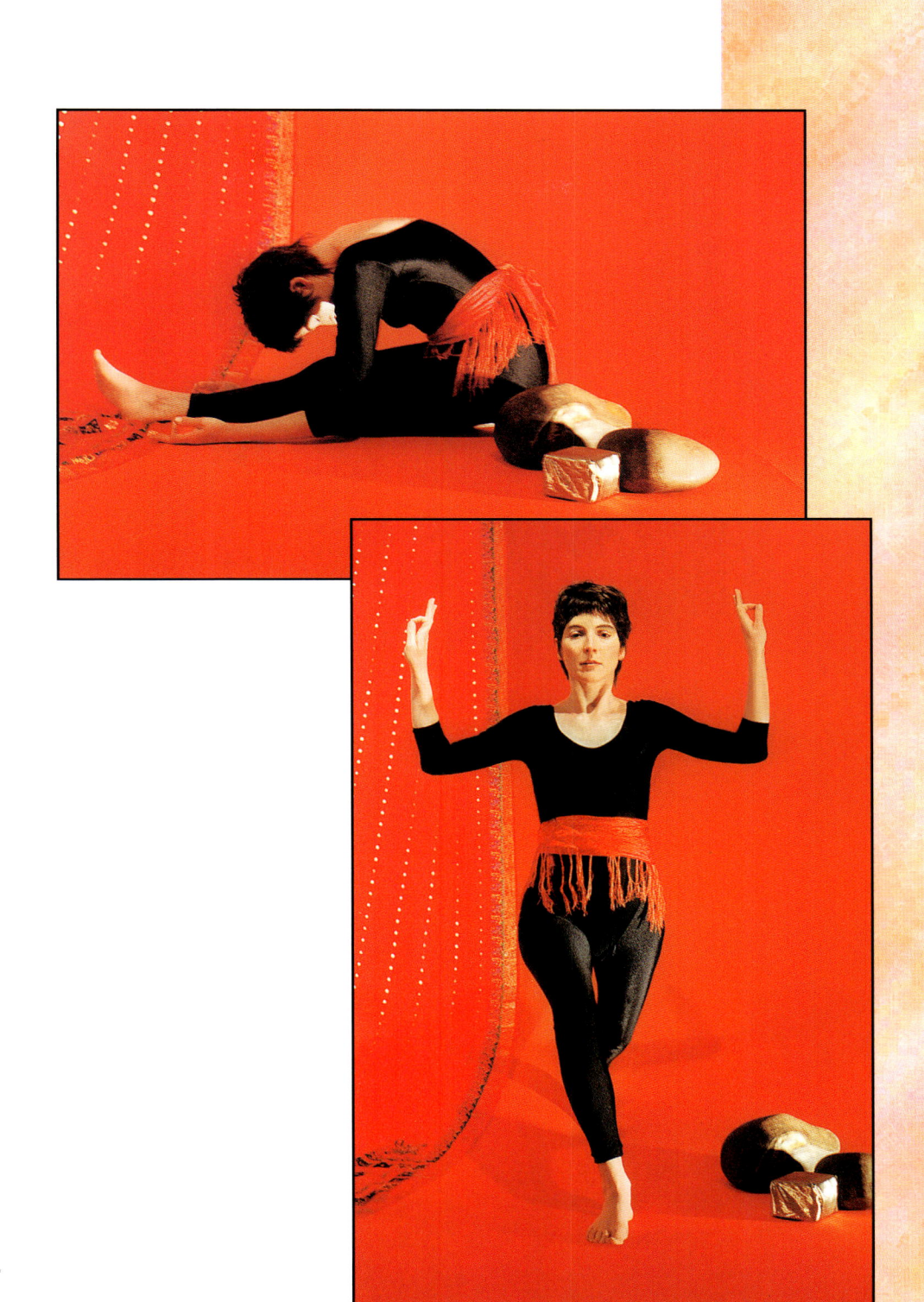

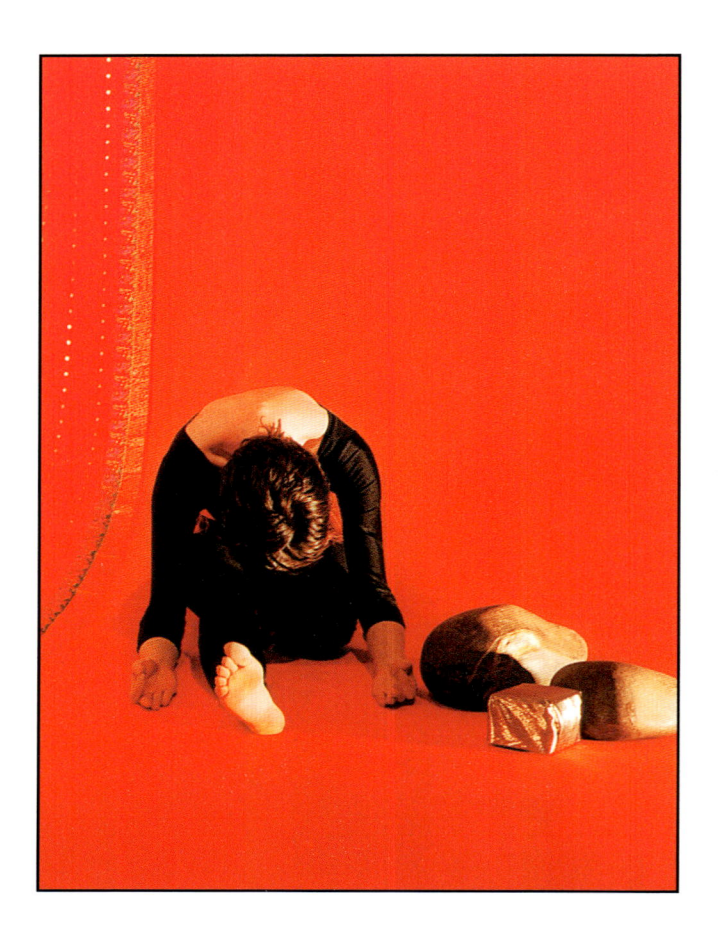

If you select a Spanish music with castanets and tambourines the earth centre dances but also it awakens the fire inside that part of the body which releases energy to move from the solar plexus, the middle, the Fire Chakra.

Many Indian and Middle Eastern musics which awaken the "gypsy within" are working on earth and fire. It encourages wondrously adventurous leaps, darting, springing, a trampoline of earth and fire, as well as standing tall and steady in one's own light and dignity.

Russian and Polish musics being from the colder climates also have lots of fire and earth.

Water music contains all the character of water, be it tiny, tinkling droplets shining in sunlight ... trickling and bouncing over rocks, splashing the ferns, flowing deep and slow, close to the earth, swirling in spiralling whirlpools, raging torrents and waterfalls. It contains the rise and fall of the ocean, the roll of waves against the shore, the thunderous crashing of a turbulent sea. A listening can become a feeling which can be expressed through movement directed from the pelvic area, from the lower back and yet guided by the hips. Flowing is the appropriate description ... whether that be flowing onwards, to and fro, rising and falling, spiralling into a whirlpool or moving gracefully like a swan drifting across a lake. Sometimes in a turbulent sense the water needs the earth and the fire too. Maybe Schubert's impromptus were written to awaken the dance of the water ... along with certain Strauss compositions, works of Smetana, Brahms, Liszt and many more.

To dance from the heart centre (the middle of the chest) is to fly like a bird, as if the legs and feet are almost non-existent or just simply an after thought that follows the movement. Consider the graceful spiralling of an eagle, the dipping and swooping of a kite, the wind whirling or softly whispering through mobiles, discovering the wings of a butterfly. Flute and oboe musics are often of the Air Chakra ... Chopin nocturnes and waltzes seem to dance in the air along with many Mozart compositions.

When the consciousness is lifted even higher perhaps with certain musics of Bach, Beethoven for instance or the haunting French composer, Debussy, we could find ourselves moving primarily from the Throat Chakra. The dancer can be inspired by the image of a transparent bubble of light, or maybe thistledown floating lighter than the air itself.

The sacred dance is experienced in a transformed state of such beauty. It is when the magic of the higher mind is awakened and it seems that each movement is pure. The essence of the dance is of a spiritual nature because it comes from the spirit within. It responds to the sound of mystical bells, choirs of angelic voices, certain sacred works of the greats, Handel, Bach, Beethoven, Albinoni, and of course the ancient temple musics of the Far East.

Yet in the wholeness we seek on the never ending journey of self awareness through yoga, the real dance is when all the centres are wide open to respond to "what is".

In other words ...

What is happening at this very moment?
What does it ask of me?
What am I feeling in response to the moment?
What quality does it awaken?

"What is" asks everything of us. It is the ultimate awareness. It demands embracing completely even if it is not to our liking. It demands trust, surrender and humility. It demands courage, self-esteem and energy. It demands gratitude, generosity, light-heartedness and enthusiasm.

It demands being totally true to oneself. It demands standing tall in your own beam of light. It demands taking full responsibility for your life, your choices, your decisions. It demands unconditional LOVE.

The yoga suggests that true happiness resides in ...

Being with "WHAT IS"
Breathing "WHAT IS"
Dancing with "WHAT IS"
Radiating "WHAT IS"
Loving "WHAT IS"

But there is nothing more beautiful than realising that no matter how far the long journey stretches out before each one of us we <u>can</u> BECOME ONE WITH "WHAT IS" !!!

Om Tat Sat
"THOU ART THAT"

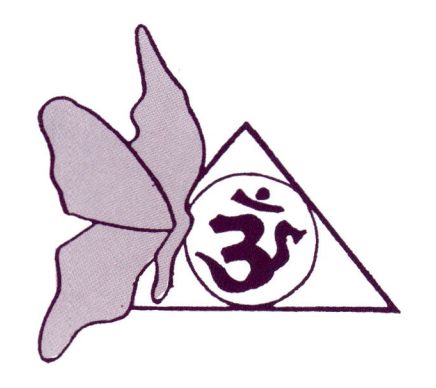